recipes for
arthritis
health

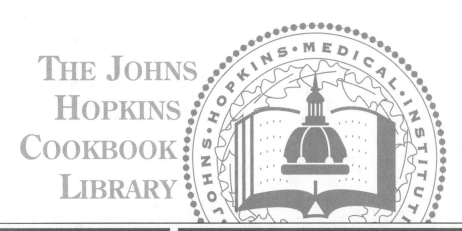

THE JOHNS HOPKINS COOKBOOK LIBRARY

recipes for arthritis health

Medical Editor

JOHN A. FLYNN, M.D., F.A.C.P., F.A.C.R.

Nutrition Editor

LORA BROWN WILDER, Sc.D., M.S., R.D.

REBUS
NEW YORK

JOHNS HOPKINS HEALTH AFTER 50 PUBLICATIONS

The Johns Hopkins Cookbook Library: Recipes for Arthritis Health is one of many indispensable medical publications for consumers from America's leading health center. We publish other comprehensive reference books, including consumer guides to drugs and medical tests; White Papers that provide in-depth reports on specific disorders such as coronary heart disease, arthritis, and diabetes; and *The Johns Hopkins Medical Letter HEALTH AFTER 50,* our monthly 8-page newsletter that presents recommendations from Hopkins experts on current medical issues that affect you.

All of our publications provide timely information—in clear, non-technical language—for everyone concerned with taking control of his or her own health. And, they all come from the century-old tradition of Johns Hopkins excellence.

For a trial subscription to our newsletter, you can call 904-446-4675 or write to Subscription Dept., Health After 50, P.O. Box 420179, Palm Coast, FL 32142.

For information on our publications—along with health and medical updates from our experts—visit our website:

www.hopkinsafter50.com

REBUS

This book is not intended as a substitute for the advice and expertise of a physician, pharmacist, or other health-care practitioner. Readers who suspect they may have specific medical problems should consult a physician about any suggestions made in this book.

Library of Congress Cataloging-in-Publication Data

Recipes for arthritis health / medical editor, John A. Flynn ; nutrition editor, Lora Brown Wilder.
p. cm. – (The Johns Hopkins cookbook library)
   Includes index.
   ISBN 0-929661-76-1
      1. Arthritis–Diet–Recipes. 2. Arthritis–Prevention. I. Flynn, John A., M.D. II. Wilder, Lora Brown. III. Series.

RC933 .R3626 2003
616.7'220654–dc21

2002036859

Printed in the United States of America
10 9 8 7 6 5 4 3 2 1

contents

eating for arthritis health

How diet affects arthritis has been a source of controversy and misinformation over the years, and has often resulted in expensive and questionable remedies and diets. Due to the scarcity of well-controlled studies, many arthritis specialists believe that there simply isn't enough reliable information to determine whether certain food constituents can cause, prevent, or ameliorate symptoms of arthritis.

Health professionals, however, encourage people with osteoarthritis or rheumatoid arthritis to achieve and maintain normal weight and maximum nutritional health by eating a variety of nutrient-dense foods such as deeply colored fruits and vegetables, legumes, whole grains, lean sources of protein, and low-fat dairy foods. In addition, because nutritional well-being can be impaired by the effects of certain arthritis medications that are taken frequently or on a long-term basis, and because the ability to absorb nutrients may be decreased by natural age-related changes, it would be a good idea to talk to your physician about the potential need for supplements.

recipes for optimum nutrition

People with arthritis are faced with a number of daily challenges that may have an adverse impact upon nutrition and diet. For example, limited mobility, stiffness, swelling, fatigue, and joint pain can prevent people from preparing and eating adequate amounts of healthful foods. The recipes in this book are designed to contribute to a varied and balanced diet, provide ample nourishment, and promote a healthy weight.

In addition, to make it easier for people with impaired mobility and fatigue, we have created dishes that can be prepared with a minimum of chopping and in a short time (or over a long period of unattended time). This has involved using many frozen or pre-chopped foods (*see "Convenience Products," page 15*); but rest assured that the nutrition in the convenience foods we have used is equal to (and sometimes superior to) the corresponding fresh foods.

osteoarthritis

Maintaining a healthy weight is key in helping to prevent osteoarthritis. In fact, obesity raises the risk of all types of arthritis (but especially osteoarthritis) by about 30% in both men and women, according to the Centers for Disease Control and Prevention. Carrying extra weight increases the pressure placed on the joints, which may cause the gradual breakdown of cartilage. Studies show that, compared with non-obese men, obese men have almost five times the risk of developing osteoarthritis of the knee, and for obese women the risk is nearly four times greater. If you are overweight, check with your physician to determine if and how you should cut back on both dietary fat and total calories.

strategies for weight loss

The good news is that even small amounts of weight loss can help to reduce the risk of developing knee osteoarthritis. And, of course, maintaining your weight at a healthy level will also help protect against the onset of other chronic conditions such as type 2 diabetes and cardiovascular disease. Always seek professional advice before embarking on a weight loss plan. In addition, be sure to speak with

WHAT TO EAT AND WHY

nutrient	food sources	health benefits
complex carbohydrates	Legumes (beans, peas), pasta, starchy vegetables (such as corn, potatoes, sweet potatoes, winter squash), whole grains	Not only do foods rich in complex carbohydrates provide a variety of vitamins, minerals, and fiber, but whole-grain varieties and legumes also are filling, which is helpful in curbing appetite. Maintaining a healthy weight may prevent osteoarthritis as well as heart disease and type 2 diabetes.
fiber	apples, barley, beans, broccoli, dried fruit, grapefruit, legumes, mushrooms, oats, pears, potatoes with their skins, whole-grain breads and cereals	People who eat fiber-rich diets get less hungry between meals, feel fuller more quickly at mealtime, and tend to consume fewer calories throughout the day. And high-fiber foods are packed with nutritional value.
calcium	bok choy, broccoli, calcium-fortified juice, canned salmon and sardines with bones, low-fat dairy foods, soybeans, tofu (that has been processed with calcium), white beans	Calcium-rich foods are necessary for bone health, which may be compromised by long-term use of steroids. Health professionals generally recommend milk and other low-fat dairy foods as a primary source of calcium because these foods offer the greatest concentration of calcium. Speak with your physician about taking a calcium and vitamin D supplement.
folate	asparagus, avocados, beans, beets, broccoli, chick-peas, oranges and orange juice, lentils, soybeans, spinach, wheat germ, fortified cereal and bread	Folate, a B vitamin that is vital for health, can be depleted in people who are taking methotrexate (a drug sometimes prescribed for rheumatoid arthritis). Speak with your physician about taking a folic acid or B-complex supplement.

eating for arthritis health

RECENT RESEARCH

DON'T SKIP BREAKFAST WHEN YOU DIET

A new study supports what nutritionists and health professionals already knew: Among a group of people who are successful at losing weight and keeping it off, most eat breakfast every day. Researchers analyzed data on 2,959 participants who were enrolled in the National Weight Control Registry, which is part of an ongoing study of adults who lost at least 30 pounds and kept the weight off for a year or more.

Results showed that 78% of the participants had breakfast 7 days a week; 5% had breakfast 6 days a week; 5% had breakfast 5 days a week; and only 4% said they never ate breakfast. The breakfast eaters reported slightly more physical activity than non-breakfast eaters.

The study participants tended to consume a diet consisting primarily of carbohydrates, with 20% to 25% of daily calories from fat. The study authors speculate that eating breakfast may reduce late-day hunger, which tends to lead to overeating. They also note that consuming nutrients at breakfast may leave people with a better ability to perform the physical activity that also promotes weight loss.

OBESITY RESEARCH
VOLUME 10, PAGE 78
FEBRUARY, 2002

your physician about exercise: Increased physical activity can help to alleviate symptoms of osteoarthritis and is also a key component of a weight-loss program.

The following nutrients may help with your weight-loss efforts:

low-fat protein Choosing protein-rich foods that are low in saturated fat will help to lower your fat and calorie intake. Good low-fat sources of protein include fish, shellfish, poultry without the skin, lean cuts of meat, egg whites, and low-fat dairy foods. Good plant sources of protein include tofu and dried beans, especially soybeans. Though both tofu and soybeans can have quite a bit of fat (and calories), they are extremely low in saturated fat. In fact, most of their fat is unsaturated and includes healthful essential fatty acids such as linoleic acid and small amounts of omega-3 fatty acids. (And reduced-fat tofu is now available on the market.)

complex carbohydrates Complex carbohydrates provide a satisfying volume of food with a minimum of calories, especially when they replace fat in the diet; they provide a feeling of fullness, which helps curb appetite; and whole-grain complex carbohydrates are generally rich in fiber, which has multiple health benefits (*see opposite*). The base of the United States Department of Agriculture (USDA) Food Guide Pyramid depicts that the bulk of what Americans should eat is foods from the complex carbohydrate group. The USDA recommends six to eleven servings of complex carbohydrates per day. For example, one serving of complex carbohydrates would be: 1 slice of bread, 1 ounce of ready-to-eat cereal, or ½ cup of cooked cereal, rice or pasta.

fiber Eating plenty of fiber-rich foods can help you maintain a proper weight. The two main types of dietary fiber—soluble and insoluble—contribute to weight control in specific ways. Soluble fiber (also called "viscous" fiber)—found in oats, barley, legumes, and dried and fresh fruit—forms a gel around food particles, which slows their passage through the stomach and delays hunger signals sent to the brain. The other type of fiber, insoluble fiber (also sometimes called "roughage") is the sponge-like form of dietary fiber found in broccoli, potatoes with their skins, apples, beans, and whole-grain breads and cereals. This type of fiber absorbs water in the digestive tract, thus supplying bulk that contributes to a feeling of fullness, which helps to discourage overeating.

In addition to its benefit to a weight loss regimen, soluble fiber helps to lower LDL cholesterol levels, while insoluble fiber is useful in preventing constipation. Most foods contain some of each type of fiber. Bulk up on both soluble and insoluble dietary fiber by consuming a variety of fruits and vegetables and a mix of whole-grain foods.

rheumatoid arthritis

People who have rheumatoid arthritis may be underweight, may suffer from nutritional deficiencies associated with certain medications (*see "Drug/Nutrient Interactions," page 10*), and are faced with the challenge of increasing both calorie and protein intake. Weight loss and increased need for protein are thought to be caused by the inflammatory substances produced by people with rheumatoid arthritis. Because these people also tend to have an increased risk for heart disease, they should take extra steps to eat a heart-smart diet that is low in saturated fat and cholesterol. Speak with your physician about your specific dietary needs.

gout

Gout is a form of arthritis caused by high blood levels of uric acid, a substance derived both from the diet and from certain metabolic processes. High levels of uric acid, which cause recurrent bouts of acute "gouty" arthritis, may occur because a person produces too much uric acid or eliminates too little in the urine. It was once believed that gout was provoked by substances called purines found in anchovies, liver, and other animal organs. Research, however, has since shown

omega-3 fatty acids in fish

Quite a bit of interest has surrounded the potential benefits of the omega-3 fatty acids found in fish. While some research indicates that these fatty acids may reduce the inflammatory process that accompanies rheumatoid arthritis, there have not been enough well-controlled studies in people that would allow health professionals to recommend supplements of these dietary fats as therapy, and so their use remains controversial. Fish oil supplements cause upset stomach and they may also cause bleeding in people who are taking warfarin (Coumadin) or nonsteroidal anti-inflammatory drugs (NSAIDs). In addition, a safe and effective dosage of omega-3s has not been determined. In the meantime, it is likely that the increased consumption of fish rich in omega-3 fatty acids (such as salmon, herring, and mackerel) will offer protection against coronary heart disease. Eating fish is also an excellent way to obtain lean protein and essential vitamins and minerals.

that avoiding purine-rich foods has little impact on blood uric acid levels. Excessive alcohol intake or fasting can raise uric acid levels and precipitate an attack of gouty arthritis.

Obesity increases the risk of developing gout; about half of patients with gout are 15% or more above their ideal weight. Preliminary research shows that some people with gout may also have an increased incidence of the metabolic syndrome, a cluster of conditions that include abdominal obesity, high triglycerides, low HDL cholesterol, high blood pressure, and impaired glucose tolerance.

drug/nutrient interactions

methotrexate & folate Methotrexate, a medication sometimes prescribed for rheumatoid arthritis, can compromise proper nutrition by depleting the body's folate stores. Vital for health, folate is a B vitamin found in many foods, including dark green leafy vegetables, citrus, and legumes. Folic acid, a man-made form of folate, is added to fortified grain foods such as bread, rolls, flour, cornmeal, rice, pasta, and ready-to-eat breakfast cereals. Because too much folate can mask symptoms of vitamin B_{12} deficiency, individuals with rheumatoid arthritis are urged to consult a physician about a B-complex supplement that contains both folic acid and B_{12}.

corticosteroids (steroids) & calcium Getting enough calcium is vital for bone health, and it's particularly important if your bones are being adversely affected by steroids, which are sometimes used to treat rheumatoid arthritis. Along with causing weight gain, the long-term use of steroids may result in rapid bone loss that leads to osteoporosis and bone fractures. Along with calcium, you also need enough vitamin D, to ensure proper calcium absorption. Speak with your physician about calcium and vitamin D supplements.

cyclosporine & grapefruit juice Grapefruit juice contains a compound that may interfere with how certain medications are metabolized in the intestine. As a result, an increased amount of the medication can be absorbed into the blood. Higher blood levels of the medication can lead to side effects. A wide range of drugs may be affected by grapefruit juice, including cyclosporine, which is sometimes prescribed for rheumatoid arthritis. To play it safe, avoid drinking grapefruit juice within several hours of taking medication; and though the fresh fruit itself may not cause a problem, it is also prudent to avoid eating grapefruit when taking medication. Talk to your pharmacist or physician if you have concerns about the effects of grapefruit.

add these foods to your diet

asparagus

what's in it Low in fat and calories, asparagus provides vitamin B_6, folate, vitamin C, niacin, riboflavin, beta carotene, and fiber. One cup of cooked asparagus will give you 263 mcg of folate, which is about 66% of the recommended daily intake for this important B vitamin.

cook's notes: To retain more of asparagus' water-soluble B vitamins, steam or microwave asparagus instead of boiling it.

barley

what's in it Barley is a rich source of complex carbohydrates and provides thiamin, niacin, vitamin B_6, iron, and zinc. Barley provides ample amounts of fiber, particularly beta glucan, a soluble fiber that helps to lower LDL cholesterol. In addition, I cup of cooked pearl barley will supply about 25% of the recommended daily intake (55 mcg) of the antioxidant mineral selenium.

cook's notes: Barley comes in various forms, including hulled, pearl (or pearled), and quick-cooking. The most nutritious of the three is hulled, because it still has its bran layer; but it can be difficult to find and takes longer to cook. Pearl barley and quick-cooking barley are nutritionally equal.

beans, dried

what's in it A nourishing, low-fat source of plant protein, dried beans are high in complex carbohydrates, fiber, B vitamins (especially folate), and minerals, such as potassium, magnesium, and selenium. Beans are particularly rich in cholesterol-lowering soluble fiber. And the insoluble fiber in dried beans helps to improve regularity by speeding the passage of food through the intestine. The ample fiber content of dried beans also bolsters weight-control efforts by contributing to a feeling of fullness.

cook's notes: The gas-causing culprits in beans are carbohydrates called oligosaccharides. Some theories suggest that presoaking beans, and then discarding the soaking water before cooking them, will get rid of some of the oligosaccharides.

berries

what's in it Not only are berries rich in fiber, vitamin C, and flavor, but they also contain phytochemicals, such as ellagic acid and anthocyanins, which are under review for the potential to prevent certain diseases. Population studies show that a high intake of fruit and vegetables may help to lower the risk for certain types of cancer and heart disease.

bok choy

what's in it One cup of cooked bok choy will give you 24% of the RDA for beta carotene, 17% of the RDA for vitamin B6, and almost half (49%) of the RDA for vitamin C. Bok choy also offers folate, calcium, fiber, and potassium. What bok choy will not give you is a lot of calories: One cup has only 20 calories.

cook's notes: Bok choy is ideally suited to stir-fries not only because of its Asian origins, but also because by cooking the bok choy in a small amount of oil, the beta carotene content of the vegetable becomes more available to the body. This quick-cooking method also helps preserve the B vitamin content, since these are water-soluble vitamins that would be reduced if you cooked the bok choy in water.

broccoli

what's in it A high-fiber, nutrient-dense food, broccoli is a good source of folate, riboflavin, vitamin B_6, vitamin C, and potassium. Noted for its wealth of phytochemicals, broccoli (and especially broccoli sprouts) is a leading source of sulforaphane, a compound that helps prevent cell damage associated with aging, cancer, and other illnesses. Broccoli also contains beta carotene and lutein, carotenoids with antioxidant properties.

cook's notes: To preserve broccoli's nutrients, cook it as briefly as possible: steam, microwave, or stir-fry it instead of boiling it. Raw broccoli has more vitamin C than cooked; however, cooking will make the carotenoids in the vegetable more bioavailable.

bulgur

what's in it Of the various forms of whole wheat, bulgur is the easiest to cook, requiring nothing more than steeping (soaking) in boiling water. And bulgur is also rich in flavor, texture, and nutritional value. Bulgur is a good source of complex carbohydrates, magnesium, iron, niacin, and fiber.

add these foods to your diet

butternut squash

what's in it The deep orange flesh of butternut squash indicates the presence of carotenoids: In fact, 1 cup of cooked, mashed butternut squash provides 93% of the RDA for the carotenoid, beta carotene. Rich in complex carbohydrates, butternut squash is a good source of dietary fiber, vitamin C, magnesium, and potassium.

cantaloupe

what's in it Low in calories and rich in potassium, vitamin B$_6$, and vitamin C, cantaloupe is an excellent source of the antioxidant beta carotene. In fact, cantaloupes provide more beta carotene than any other melon. The body converts beta carotene into vitamin A, which is important for eye health and for promoting healthy cell growth.

cook's notes: Make sure to wash the rinds of cantaloupe (as well as other melons), since they are susceptible to bacterial contamination because they grow on the ground. To preserve a cantaloupe's nutritional content, it is a good idea to buy whole cantaloupes rather than pre-cut halves or cubes. When exposed to air the vitamin C becomes diminished.

corn

what's in it A highly popular food, complex carbohydrate-rich corn provides rich texture and flavor. Most varieties are good sources of fiber, thiamin, folate, potassium, iron, and magnesium. Only yellow corn, however, contains beta carotene as well as the carotenoids lutein and zeaxanthin. These two carotenoids are associated with healthy eyes and may be helpful in preventing cataracts and age-related macular degeneration.

cook's notes: To preserve the water-soluble B vitamins in fresh corn (folate and thiamin), it's best to steam rather than boil it. If this isn't practical (since most people cook corn-on-the-cob by the dozen), then be sure to cook for no longer than 10 minutes in boiling water to minimize nutrient loss.

dairy

what's in it Low-fat (1%) or fat-free (also called skim) milk and yogurt provide high-quality protein, calcium, B vitamins (especially vitamin B12), and minerals, without the added saturated fat, which has more calories and increases harmful LDL cholesterol (1% milk has a small amount of saturated fat but much less than whole milk). For the most calcium per cup, fat-free plain yogurt is the best, at 488 mg (about 40% of the recommended daily intake). After that, in descending order, are low-fat yogurt (448 mg), fat-free milk (352 mg), and 1% milk (300 mg), all excellent sources of calcium.

fish, fatty

what's in it All fish are an excellent source of lean protein, vitamins B$_6$, B$_{12}$, E, and niacin, as well as selenium and iron. And fatty fish such as salmon, mackerel, tuna, herring, and sardines are particularly notable for their rich supply of heart-healthy fats called omega-3 fatty acids. In fact, they are so beneficial for cardiovascular health that the American Heart Association recommends that people eat two servings of fatty fish a week to prevent heart disease. It is believed that omega-3 fatty acids help lower the risk of developing an irregular heart rhythm that can cause fatal heart attacks. These fats may also help reduce blood clotting. Exactly how omega-3 fatty acids yield these benefits is under investigation. And while fatty fish do contain moderate amounts of dietary cholesterol, they are low in saturated fats, which are more of a health risk than dietary cholesterol. Canned salmon and sardines, with the bones, are also a good source of calcium.

cook's notes: Cooking fish destroys the parasites and potentially harmful microorganisms that are present in raw fish.

grains, whole

what's in it Whole-grain foods such as whole-grain breads, brown rice, and oatmeal, are high in fiber and provide complex carbohydrates, folate, riboflavin, thiamin, niacin, iron, zinc, magnesium, selenium, and vitamin E. Studies have shown that whole-grain foods help to lower the risk of type 2 diabetes and cardiovascular disease. Whole grains retain their bran (the fiber-rich outer layer of the grain) and the germ (the nutrient-dense inner part), which provide nutrients and phytochemicals. Wheat germ, for example, offers folate, thiamin, magnesium, vitamin B$_6$, iron, selenium, vitamin E, zinc, and fiber. It is also rich in polyunsaturated fats. Wheat bran, the outer layer of the wheat kernel, provides fiber, B vitamins, protein, and iron. The Food Guide Pyramid recommends that adults eat 6 to 11 servings of grain foods daily; several of those servings should be whole grains. Look for products with "whole grain" or "100 percent whole wheat" at the top of the ingredient list to make sure you are buying whole-grain foods. High-fiber whole grains are heart-healthy and they are also helpful in weight loss.

add these foods to your diet

cook's notes: Because the germ of whole grains contains oil, whole-grain products should be refrigerated to prevent them from turning rancid.

lentils

what's in it An inexpensive, low-fat source of fiber, potassium, and zinc, the lentil is also a good source of B vitamins, including folate. For example, a mere 1/2-cup serving of lentils will supply almost half of your daily requirement for this B vitamin. Plant protein and complex carbohydrates are also supplied by lentils, which have provided sustenance for people for thousands of years.

cook's notes: To protect the water-soluble vitamins folate and vitamin B_6, don't cook lentils in too much water; and if any cooking liquid needs to be drained off, try to use it in the recipe or save for soups or other dishes. Soluble fiber in lentils is made more bioavailable as the lentils cook and the fiber dissolves (this also softens the lentils). Eat foods high in vitamin C along with lentils to enhance iron absorption.

lima beans

what's in it Lima beans are a good source of B vitamins (vitamin B_6, niacin, folate), fiber (especially soluble fiber in the form of pectin), iron, potassium, and magnesium; and they have very little fat.

cook's notes: Lima beans are available fresh (rare), frozen, and dried. All three forms of the bean are good sources of nutrients, but some water-soluble B vitamins will be lost when the limas are cooked in water. Use as little water as possible (or steam fresh or frozen beans), and try to

incorporate the cooking water into the dish. Cooking limas in soup is a good solution.

oranges

what's in it While most people tend to associate the benefits of oranges and their juice with vitamin C, they may not be aware that oranges are also a rich source of folate, potassium, fiber, and thiamin. While 1 cup of orange juice supplies 91% of the suggested daily intake for vitamin C, the whole fruit offers the added benefit of more than 3 grams of fiber.

potatoes

what's in it Rich in complex carbohydrates, vitamin C, thiamin, iron, niacin, and fiber, potatoes also supply ample amounts of potassium. Low in calories, rich in nutrients, potatoes are an ideal food for people who are watching their weight. In addition, one large baked potato gives you almost 50% of the recommended daily intake of vitamin B_6.

cook's notes: Try to eat potatoes with the skin, where most of the iron and fiber are found. And if you boil potatoes, leave the skin on (even if you're peeling them after cooking) and try to reuse the cooking water, where many of the B vitamins wind up.

rice, brown

what's in it A nutritious whole grain, brown rice has only the outer hull removed, which means that it retains—along with its bran layer—thiamin, niacin, vitamin B_6, and small amounts of vitamin E. And because the bran is not milled away, brown rice provides four times more insoluble fiber than white rice.

soybeans

Compared with other legumes, soybeans are a complete source of protein since they have all the essential amino acids required for the building and maintenance of human body tissues. Studies show that when substituted for animal protein in the diet, soy protein helps to reduce LDL cholesterol and triglycerides without having an adverse effect on the beneficial HDL cholesterol.

tofu

what's in it Tofu is highly nutritious and, when substituted for saturated fats, is a heart-healthy food that offers a wide range of nutrients. In addition to soy protein and phytochemicals called isoflavones, tofu has magnesium, selenium, and zinc. And the type of tofu made with a calcium salt (check the label to be sure) can also contribute to your calcium needs.

turkey

what's in it Turkey is an excellent source of protein, riboflavin, niacin, vitamin B_6, vitamin B_{12}, selenium, iron, and zinc. While most of the fat in turkey is found in the skin, turkey meat is so low in fat that eating 3 ounces of roasted breast meat with skin would furnish only 130 calories, 19% of them coming from fat. The dark meat is higher in fat than the light meat, but it is still relatively lean if eaten without the skin.

cook's notes: Although less fatty than chicken, turkey skin still has a substantial amount of fat. For roasting whole turkey or turkey breast, you can leave the skin on, but remove it before eating.

recipes: a user's guide

▶ focus on food, not numbers

The basic message, regardless of health concerns, is to eat a variety of foods, especially fruits, vegetables, and grains, with a minimum of fat (specifically saturated fat). If you follow these precepts, you probably will not have to concern yourself with fat and calorie calculations. (Note that your calorie needs are determined by a host of factors including body mass, how much you exercise on a regular basis, and such biological factors as metabolism and genetics.) However, if you are trying to keep track, the most important thing to understand is that you should be evaluating your intake not for an individual dish in a meal, and not even for the meal itself, but for a day's intake—and, ideally, for a week's intake.

▶ nutrition analysis

Each recipe in this cookbook is accompanied by a nutritional analysis, including values for calories, total fat (with the amount of saturated fat in parenthesis), cholesterol, dietary fiber, carbohydrates, protein, and sodium. "Number crunchers" will want to use the actual values to determine their day's intake, but almost all of the recipes are designed to conform to sensible intakes of calories and fat (see "On the Menu," opposite page).

▶ good source of

In the nutritional analysis for each recipe is a section called "good source of," which lists vitamins, minerals, and other healthful compounds. In order for a recipe to qualify as a "good source of" a nutrient, it must provide a certain percentage of the recommended daily intake for that nutrient (when there are different values for men and women—see the chart on page 153—our calculations

are based on the higher of the two). In the case of a main-course dish, it must provide at least 25% of the recommended intake. Side dishes and desserts must provide between 10% and 20%, depending on their calories (the more calories a dish brings with it, the greater our expectation for its nutrient content).

▶ leading sources

In the back of the book, on page 152, you'll find charts that list the "Leading Sources" of the nutrients featured in this book. A food makes it onto the chart by having at least 10% of the recommended intake for that nutrient (see the chart on page 153). Knowing which foods are especially high in important nutrients should help you when you are choosing foods to cook as side dishes, or even creating your own recipes.

▶ spotlite recipes

In our "Spotlite" recipes, we focus on certain aspects of cooking that we think can make healthful eating more enjoyable or more efficient—or both. A "Spotlite" recipe can focus on a healthy cooking technique, unusual ingredients, or a health makeover. Here's what you'll find in these pages:

- **Sweet Potato & Baked Ham Salad with Ginger Dressing** (page 65), an introduction to a great new ingredient, ginger juice.
- **Broiled Five-Spice Chicken** (page 80), using a Chinese spice blend called five-spice powder.
- **Roast Turkey Reuben** (page 84), an American classic gets a makeover.
- **Mediterranean Peas & Cheese Salad** (page 88), the benefits of the layered salad.

▶ crockpot cooking

There is a collection of recipes in the book created for the electric slow cooker, which is designed for hands-off cooking. For homey dishes such as soups and stews, all you have to do (more or less) is throw the ingredients into the pot, turn on the cooker, and let it simmer gently for a couple of hours. This can be important for anyone who does not want to be on his or her feet for any length of time.

▶ off-the-shelf recipes

With these recipes we try to take advantage of packaged foods without compromising the healthful nature of the dish. Since cooking from scratch takes time and fast food is often bad for your health, we've tried to find a satisfying middle ground.

▶ in the margins

On most recipe pages, you'll find tips that fall into one of the following categories:

F.Y.I. This is additional information on an ingredient in a dish or the nutrient content of a dish. For example, if the nutrition analysis tells you that the dish is a "good source of" folate, the F.Y.I. will explain which ingredients are providing the folate, and also remind you what folate is good for.

ON THE Menu If the fat or calories in an individual dish are a bit high, On the Menu will suggest other dishes that will create a well-rounded meal and also keep the overall fat percentage of that meal at a reasonable level. It's important to understand that a dish should fit into the context of a full meal and not be evaluated on its own.

KITCHEN tip Kitchen tips are, as the title suggests, information of value to the cook: how to shop for certain ingredients, short-cuts to make the recipe easier, or an explanation of a technique used in the recipe.

convenience products

Wherever possible, we have called for ingredients that exist in frozen, canned, or pre-cut versions to reduce wear and tear on the fingers and hands of the cook. (In the case of frozen vegetables, the nutritional value is comparable—or superior—to that of fresh produce, because vegetables to be frozen are processed immediately after picking.) Here are some convenience foods that we used in our recipes and that can be found in supermarkets nationwide. The list doesn't include the more obvious products, such as canned tomatoes or frozen peas.

- minced fresh ginger
- minced fresh garlic (note that you should buy water-packed, not oil-packed)
- jarred chopped fresh basil
- frozen chopped onions, bell peppers
- frozen cubes of winter squash, potatoes
- mixed salad greens (there's a world of choices in this category)
- pre-sliced fresh mushrooms, onions, kale, collard greens, carrots ("chips")
- shredded fresh carrots, cabbage, broccoli, coleslaw mixture
- chicken, pork, or beef, cut for stir-fry or kebabs

Tomato & Mozzarella Salad

This quick salad can be served on its own or used as a topping for pizza or pasta. The garlic-basil dressing can be made well ahead of time and stored in a screwtop jar in the refrigerator.

per serving	
calories	154
total fat	2.8g
saturated fat	0.4g
cholesterol	5mg
dietary fiber	3g
carbohydrate	13g
protein	18g
sodium	836mg

good source of: calcium, riboflavin, vitamin B$_{12}$, vitamin C, zinc

½ cup fresh basil leaves
2 cloves garlic, peeled
2 tablespoons balsamic vinegar
2 tablespoons water
2 teaspoons olive oil
½ teaspoon salt
2 pints grape tomatoes
8 ounces shredded fat-free mozzarella

1 In a mini food processor, combine the basil, garlic, vinegar, water, oil, and salt, and puree. Transfer the dressing to a large bowl.

2 Add the tomatoes and mozzarella to the dressing, and toss to coat. Serve at room temperature or chilled. ***Makes 4 servings***

Mexican Tomato & Cheese Salad Add ½ pickled jalapeño pepper to the dressing ingredients in step 1. Substitute shredded Monterey jack cheese for the mozzarella.

Quick Pickled Vegetables

Serve these as part of an antipasto platter along with small rounds of part-skim mozzarella and crusty bread. You could also serve the vegetables as a simple side dish for cold poached chicken or grilled flank steak.

¾ cup dry white wine
¾ cup water
½ teaspoon basil
¼ teaspoon crushed red pepper flakes
¾ teaspoon salt
8 ounces peeled baby carrots
1 package (10 ounces) frozen cauliflower florets
1 package (10 ounces) frozen Italian green beans
¼ cup white wine vinegar
2 teaspoons olive oil

1   In a large skillet, bring the wine, water, basil, red pepper flakes, and ¼ teaspoon of the salt to a simmer. Add the carrots, cover, and cook 7 minutes.

2 Add the cauliflower and beans. Return to a simmer and cook, uncovered, until the carrots are crisp-tender, about 5 minutes.

3 Transfer the vegetables and cooking liquid to a medium bowl. Stir in the vinegar, oil, and remaining ½ teaspoon salt. Cover and refrigerate for at least 4 hours or overnight. Serve the vegetables chilled or at room temperature. *Makes 4 servings*

Balsamic Vegetables Substitute balsamic vinegar for the white wine vinegar. Use 2 cups chopped green pepper instead of cauliflower, and 1 package (10 ounces) frozen corn kernels instead of green beans.

F.Y.I.

This antipasto is similar to Italian pickled vegetables called *giardiniera*. The word *giardiniera* means "gardener," and the pickles can be any combination of vegetables, though they most typically include cauliflower, probably because the florets are so sturdy.

per serving	
calories	237
total fat	2g
saturated fat	0.6g
cholesterol	12mg
dietary fiber	2g
carbohydrate	54g
protein	6g
sodium	328mg

good source of: niacin, potassium, thiamin, vitamin B$_6$, vitamin C

Black Forest Ham & Melon

The honey-lime dressing brings out the sweetness of the melon and provides a nice counterpoint to the saltiness of the ham.

8 wedges (1 inch wide) honeydew melon, rind removed
3 ounces very thinly sliced Black Forest or other smoked ham
⅓ cup honey
¼ cup lime juice
½ teaspoon pepper

1 Divide the melon among 4 serving plates and drape the ham over the melon.

2 In a small bowl, whisk together the honey, lime juice, and pepper. Spoon the dressing over the melon and serve. ***Makes 4 servings***

Smoked Turkey & Cantaloupe Thinly sliced smoked turkey makes a good substitute for smoked ham. Use cantaloupe instead of honeydew. Add 2 teaspoons of Dijon mustard to the dressing.

Spicy Black Bean Dip

While this scrumptious dip is slightly spicy, you'll want to add more cayenne if you're a big fan of spicy food.

2 cans (15½ ounces each) black beans, rinsed and
    drained
½ cup water
3 tablespoons distilled white vinegar
2 tablespoons lemon juice
2½ teaspoons cumin
1½ teaspoons garlic powder
1½ teaspoons coriander
¾ teaspoon salt
½ teaspoon cayenne pepper

In a food processor, combine all of the ingredients and pulse until well combined but with some texture remaining. *Makes 3 cups*

Curried White Bean Dip Omit the coriander and cayenne and use 2 teaspoons of curry powder instead. Substitute canned cannellini beans for the black beans.

per ⅓ cup	
calories	75
total fat	0.5g
saturated fat	0.1g
cholesterol	0mg
dietary fiber	5g
carbohydrate	14g
protein	5g
sodium	351mg

good source of: fiber, folate, magnesium, thiamin

Cheese-Stuffed Portobellos

The creamy base for the cheese in these stuffed mushrooms is created by an unexpected (but healthful) ingredient: cream of rice. Its smooth texture helps give the impression that you are getting more cheese than you actually are (a good thing, healthwise!). You can find dried grated orange zest in the spice aisle.

4 portobello mushrooms (4 ounces each)
3 tablespoons cream of rice
¾ cup water
3 tablespoons chopped sun-dried tomatoes
   (not oil-packed)
½ cup shredded fat-free mozzarella cheese
2 tablespoons grated Parmesan cheese
¼ teaspoon salt
¼ teaspoon grated orange peel, fresh or dried

1 Preheat the oven to 450°F. Remove and discard the stems from the mushrooms. Place the mushroom caps, gill-side down, in a baking pan large enough to hold them in a single layer. Add enough water to just cover the bottom of the pan. Cover and bake until the mushrooms are tender, about 10 minutes. Discard any liquid remaining in the pan. Leave the oven on.

2 Meanwhile, in a small bowl, stir the cream of rice into the ¾ cup of water until smooth. Let stand until thick, about 5 minutes.

3 Stir in the sun-dried tomatoes, ¼ cup of the mozzarella, the Parmesan, salt, and orange zest.

4 Turn the mushrooms gill-side up and spoon the cream of rice mixture into the cavities. Sprinkle the remaining ¼ cup of mozzarella over the top. Bake, uncovered, until the cheese has melted and the mixture is piping hot, about 10 minutes. *Makes 4 servings*

per mushroom	
calories	87
total fat	1g
saturated fat	0.6g
cholesterol	5mg
dietary fiber	3g
carbohydrate	12g
protein	9g
sodium	314mg

good source of: calcium, fiber

F.Y.I.

Mushrooms provide riboflavin, niacin, vitamin B_6, and a type of soluble fiber called beta-glucan. And as a boon to those watching their calorie intake, mushrooms have a satisfying flavor and texture for almost no calories (2 cups of raw mushrooms have only about 40 calories).

Two-Bean & Sausage Soup

<table>
<tr><td colspan="2">per serving</td></tr>
<tr><td>calories</td><td>359</td></tr>
<tr><td>total fat</td><td>12g</td></tr>
<tr><td>saturated fat</td><td>3.5g</td></tr>
<tr><td>cholesterol</td><td>72mg</td></tr>
<tr><td>dietary fiber</td><td>12g</td></tr>
<tr><td>carbohydrate</td><td>42g</td></tr>
<tr><td>protein</td><td>22g</td></tr>
<tr><td>sodium</td><td>920mg</td></tr>
</table>

good source of: fiber, folate, magnesium, potassium, thiamin, vitamin B_6, vitamin C, zinc

ON THE *Menu*

To round out the meal, serve a salad of mixed greens with a low-fat red wine vinaigrette and whole-grain rolls. For dessert, have Baked Bananas (page 129) with fat-free vanilla yogurt dolloped on top.

Here's a hearty soup that takes only 15 minutes to put together. If you're not a fan of lima beans, use a 15-ounce can of black beans (rinsed and drained) instead.

2 teaspoons olive oil
1 cup chopped onion
2 teaspoons minced garlic
1 cup chicken broth
1 cup water
1 can (15 ounces) diced tomatoes
1 can (15 ounces) cannellini beans, rinsed and drained
1 package (10 ounces) frozen baby lima beans
6 ounces hot Italian-style turkey sausage
2 tablespoons grated Parmesan cheese

1 In a large nonstick saucepan, heat the oil over medium heat. Add the onion and garlic, and cook, stirring occasionally, until the onion is tender, about 5 minutes.

2 Add the broth, water, tomatoes, cannellini beans, and lima beans. Cover and bring to a boil over medium heat. Reduce to a simmer. Add the sausage, cover, and simmer until the sausage is cooked through and the lima beans are tender, about 10 minutes.

3 Remove the sausage and thinly slice. Ladle the soup into bowls. Add the sausage slices and sprinkle with the Parmesan. *Makes 4 servings*

Spinach, Chick-Pea & Macaroni Soup

Chick-peas add a sturdy texture and hearty flavor to this meatless soup. For a completely vegetarian soup, use vegetable broth instead of chicken broth. A squeeze of fresh lemon juice at serving time adds a fresh, sprightly flavor.

per serving	
calories	228
total fat	7.4g
saturated fat	1.2g
cholesterol	3mg
dietary fiber	8g
carbohydrate	33g
protein	10g
sodium	710mg

good source of: beta carotene, fiber, folate, magnesium, potassium, riboflavin, selenium, thiamin, vitamin B_6, vitamin C

1 tablespoon olive oil
¾ cup chopped onions
¾ cup shredded carrots
2 teaspoons minced garlic
2 cups chicken broth
1½ cups water
1 can (15½ ounces) chick-peas, rinsed and drained
¼ teaspoon salt
½ cup small pasta shapes, such as small bow-ties
    or elbows
1 package (10 ounces) frozen chopped spinach, thawed
Lemon wedges, for serving

1 In a large nonstick saucepan, heat the oil over medium heat. Add the onions, carrots, and garlic, and cook, stirring occasionally, until the onions are softened, about 7 minutes.

2 Add the broth, water, chick-peas, and salt, and bring to a boil. Add the pasta and spinach. Cover and cook until the pasta is tender, 7 to 10 minutes. Serve with lemon wedges. *Makes 4 servings*

Kale, White Bean & Macaroni Soup Substitute chopped red peppers for the carrots, cannellini beans for the chick-peas, and chopped frozen kale for the spinach.

Crockpot cooking

Two early American traditions come together in this slow-cooked recipe: succotash and chowder. Succotash is a mixture of corn and lima beans and comes from the Naragansett Indian word *msickquatash*, which means "boiled corn." Chowder comes from the French word *chaudière* and refers to the pot in which this thick stew was traditionally cooked. A classic chowder is, of course, made with seafood, but we've borrowed the concept and used chicken instead. And for some extra color, as well as healthful carotenoids, we've added diced tomatoes and shredded carrots.

Chicken & Succotash Chowder

1 package (10 ounces) frozen lima beans
1 package (10 ounces) frozen corn kernels
1½ cups chicken broth
1½ cups water
1 can (14½ ounces) diced tomatoes with basil
¾ teaspoon salt
½ teaspoon rosemary, minced
½ pound skinless, boneless chicken thighs, cut into bite-size pieces
1 cup chopped onion
1 cup chopped green bell pepper
2 teaspoons minced garlic
1 cup shredded carrots

1 Place the lima beans and corn in a 4- or 6-quart electric slow cooker. Pour the broth and water on top to help them thaw. Pour the diced tomatoes on top. Sprinkle with the salt and rosemary, and stir to combine.

2 Stir in the chicken, onion, bell pepper, garlic, and carrots. Cover and cook on low until the vegetables are tender and the chicken is cooked through, 6 to 8 hours. ***Makes 6 servings***

PER SERVING 189 calories, 3.2g total fat (0.8g saturated), 33mg cholesterol, 6g dietary fiber, 29g carbohydrate, 14g protein, 727mg sodium
Good source of: beta carotene, fiber, niacin, potassium, selenium, vitamin B$_6$, vitamin C

Creamy Winter Vegetable Stew

Just a touch of maple syrup brings out the sweetness in the winter squash and rutabaga, two root vegetables with a good amount of beta carotene.

per serving	
calories	166
total fat	2.4g
saturated fat	0.8g
cholesterol	4mg
dietary fiber	3g
carbohydrate	33g
protein	6g
sodium	364mg

good source of: beta carotene, calcium, potassium, riboflavin, vitamin C

1 teaspoon olive oil
⅓ cup chopped onions
2 cups frozen rutabaga (yellow turnip) chunks, thawed
¼ cup water
1 package (10 ounces) frozen pureed winter squash, thawed
¾ cup evaporated low-fat (2%) milk
2 tablespoons maple syrup
½ teaspoon salt

1 In a large nonstick saucepan, heat the oil over medium heat. Add the onions and cook, stirring occasionally, until tender, about 7 minutes.

2 Add the rutabaga chunks and water, and cook until the rutabaga is heated through, about 3 minutes.

3 Stir in the winter squash puree, evaporated milk, maple syrup, and salt. Cover and simmer 5 minutes to blend the flavors. ***Makes 4 servings***

Pumpkin & Black Bean Stew Omit step 2 and the rutabaga. In step 3, add the ¼ cup water and 1 can (15½ ounces) rinsed and drained black beans to the soup. Instead of winter squash, use 1 can (15 ounces) unsweetened pumpkin puree. Stir in ¼ cup of grated Parmesan cheese just before serving.

F.Y.I.

Rich in complex carbohydrates, rutabagas supply good amounts of both insoluble and cholesterol-lowering soluble fiber. These sweet, yellow-fleshed turnips also contain potassium and vitamin C: One cup of fresh rutabaga cubes provides over 35% of the daily requirement for this vitamin.

Off-the-Shelf

Between the ingredients **sitting** in your pantry and those things you are likely to have in the freezer (like chopped onion), you could have this soup on the table in about 25 minutes. While the soup is simmering, toast some whole-grain bread to go with it. If you have a hand blender, use it in step 3 instead of a food processor to puree the soup right in the saucepan.

Creamed Corn & Broccoli Soup

1 teaspoon olive oil
½ cup chopped onion
1 package (10 ounces) frozen chopped broccoli
1 can (15 ounces) no-salt-added creamed corn
1 cup chicken broth
1 cup water
½ teaspoon salt
½ teaspoon tarragon
⅛ teaspoon cayenne pepper
1 cup frozen corn kernels, thawed

1 In a large nonstick saucepan, heat the oil over medium heat. Add the onion and cook until tender, about 5 minutes.

2 Stir in the broccoli, creamed corn, broth, water, salt, tarragon, and cayenne. Bring to a boil. Reduce to a simmer, cover, and cook until the broccoli is tender, about 5 minutes.

3 Transfer the soup to a food processor and puree. Return the puree to the pan. Add the corn kernels and cook over low heat until the corn is heated through, about 3 minutes. ***Makes 4 servings***

PER SERVING 159 calories, 3.1g total fat (0.6g saturated), 1mg cholesterol, 5g dietary fiber, 33g carbohydrate, 6g protein, 563mg sodium
Good source of: fiber, folate, vitamin B_6, vitamin C

Chicken & Green Chili Soup

Here's a great recipe to turn to when you've got to pull dinner together in under half an hour. The soup itself takes only about 15 minutes, but it would be good served with a simple tossed salad and some storebought cornbread (heat it up in the oven).

per serving	
calories	225
total fat	5.5g
saturated fat	2.1g
cholesterol	42mg
dietary fiber	7g
carbohydrate	22g
protein	22g
sodium	885mg

good source of: fiber, niacin, vitamin B_6

2 cups chicken broth
½ cup water
1 can (15½ ounces) kidney beans, rinsed and drained
1 can (14½ ounces) no-salt-added stewed tomatoes
1 can (4 ounces) chopped mild green chilies
1 tablespoon chili powder
1 teaspoon minced garlic
½ pound skinless, boneless chicken breast, cut for stir-fry
¼ cup shredded Monterey jack cheese

1   In a large saucepan, stir together the broth, water, kidney beans, tomatoes, chilies, chili powder, and garlic. Cover and bring to a boil over high heat.

2   Add the chicken, reduce the heat to medium-low, cover, and simmer until the chicken is cooked through, about 5 minutes. Serve the soup topped with the cheese. *Makes 4 servings*

Spicy Pork & Pinto Soup Use pinto beans instead of kidney beans, and 1 can (14½ ounces) of diced tomatoes with jalapeño instead of the stewed tomatoes. Substitute pork loin cut for stir-fry for the chicken, and pepper jack instead of regular jack cheese.

Hearty Greens & Beans Soup

Just a small amount of turkey sausage goes a long way toward giving this kale and pinto bean soup a sense of heartiness. Instead of kale, try using chopped collards or mustard greens.

per serving	
calories	192
total fat	5.7g
saturated fat	1.4g
cholesterol	23mg
dietary fiber	8g
carbohydrate	24g
protein	13g
sodium	737mg

good source of: beta carotene, fiber, folate, potassium, vitamin C, vitamin K

1 teaspoon olive oil
1 cup chopped onion
1 teaspoon minced garlic
2 Italian-style turkey sausage links, quartered crosswise (4 ounces total)
1 can (15½ ounces) pinto beans, rinsed and drained
1 cup chicken broth
2 cups water
2 tablespoons tomato paste
½ teaspoon pepper
1 package (10 ounces) frozen chopped kale, thawed
1 tablespoon red wine vinegar

1 In a nonstick Dutch oven, heat the oil over medium heat. Add the onion and garlic, and cook, stirring occasionally, until the onion is tender, about 7 minutes.

2 Add the sausage and cook until nicely browned, about 5 minutes.

3 Add the beans, broth, water, tomato paste, and pepper, and bring to a boil. Add the kale, reduce to a simmer, cover, and cook until the kale is tender, about 10 minutes.

4 Stir in the vinegar. ***Makes 4 servings***

F.Y.I.

In most ways, Italian-style turkey sausage is similar to Italian pork sausage. The seasonings used are pretty much the same (fennel in "sweet" sausage, plus red pepper flakes for the "hot" type) and they look much alike. The big difference is in their fat content: Turkey sausages are about 75% lower in fat.

Crockpot cooking

Cabbage, Beef & Vegetable Soup

All the flavors of a hearty Middle European dish—cabbage, dill, and beef—blend together in this slow-cooked soup. The soup will be ready after as little as 4 hours, but if you want to start this in the morning to be ready for an early dinner, you can leave the soup cooking for up to 8 hours.

2 cans (14½ ounces each) no-salt-added stewed tomatoes
1¼ cups water
1 cup chicken broth
1 can (15½ ounces) cannellini beans, rinsed and drained
3 tablespoons lemon juice
1 tablespoon sugar
1 teaspoon salt
2 teaspoons minced garlic
1 package (16 ounces) coleslaw mixture
¾ pound well-trimmed beef sirloin, cut for stir-fry
1½ teaspoons dillweed
6 tablespoons reduced-fat sour cream

1 In a 4- or 6-quart electric slow cooker, combine the stewed tomatoes, water, broth, beans, lemon juice, sugar, salt, and garlic, stirring until well combined.

2 Stir in the coleslaw mixture, beef, and dillweed. Cover and cook on low for 4 to 6 hours, or until the cabbage and beef are tender.

3 Serve the soup topped with a dollop of sour cream. *Makes 4 servings*

PER SERVING 227 calories, 4.4g total fat (2g saturated), 40mg cholesterol, 7g dietary fiber, 27g carbohydrate, 19g protein, 754mg sodium
Good source of: beta carotene, folate, niacin, potassium, riboflavin, vitamin B_{12}, vitamin B_6, vitamin C, zinc

Gingered Tomato-Carrot Rice Soup

If you have a local Chinese restaurant, see if they will sell you an order of cooked rice. It's a good thing to have around, and you can keep the rice frozen.

per serving	
calories	199
total fat	3.4g
saturated fat	0.5g
cholesterol	0mg
dietary fiber	4g
carbohydrate	38g
protein	4g
sodium	714mg

good source of: potassium, selenium, vitamin C

2 teaspoons olive oil
½ cup chopped onion
1 can (14½ ounces) stewed tomatoes
1½ cups carrot juice
½ cup orange juice
1 teaspoon ground ginger
¾ teaspoon salt
2 cups cooked brown or white rice

1 In a large saucepan, heat the oil over medium heat. Add the onion and cook, stirring occasionally, until tender, about 5 minutes.

2 Add the stewed tomatoes, carrot juice, orange juice, ginger, and salt, and bring to a boil. Reduce to a simmer, cover, and cook for 5 minutes to blend the flavors.

3 Stir in the rice and serve. ***Makes 4 servings***

Shrimp, Tomato & Rice Soup For a main course, add 1 can (8 ounces) drained sliced water chestnuts and ¾ pound shelled and deveined medium shrimp to the soup for the final 5 minutes of cooking in step 2.

Off-the-Shelf

Start with a can of **tomato soup** and end up with something far more interesting than the usual back-of-the-box recipe. It just takes a couple of subtle additions, such as clam juice, roasted peppers, and sherry, to disguise the soup's humble origins. The final touch is the addition of some shredded "crab," otherwise known as surimi. Surimi is ground-up fish (usually a mild, white fish such as pollock) that is flavored and then re-shaped to resemble crabmeat. Offer a basket of crisp oyster crackers to go with the soup.

Tomato-"Crab" Bisque

1 can (10¾ ounces) reduced-fat, reduced-sodium tomato soup
¾ cup bottled clam juice
½ cup jarred roasted yellow or red peppers
½ teaspoon thyme
½ teaspoon black pepper
¼ teaspoon salt
¾ cup evaporated low-fat (2%) milk
3 ounces surimi (imitation crab), shredded
2 tablespoons sherry

1 In a medium saucepan, bring the tomato soup, clam juice, roasted pepper, thyme, black pepper, and salt to a simmer. Cover and cook 5 minutes to blend the flavors.

2 Add the evaporated milk and surimi and simmer until the surimi is heated through, about 1 minute. Stir in the sherry and serve. ***Makes 4 servings***

PER SERVING 135 calories, 2.3g total fat (1g saturated), 8mg cholesterol, 1g dietary fiber, 20g carbohydrate, 7g protein, 841mg sodium
Good source of: calcium, omega-3 fatty acids, riboflavin, selenium, vitamin B_{12}, vitamin C

Quick Black Bean Soup

If you have a hand blender, you could use it in step 3 to puree some of the beans in the soup. Pureeing only half the beans thickens the broth but still leaves the soup chunky. Add a handful of low-fat, baked tortilla chips for a flavorful, crunchy topping.

per serving	
calories	154
total fat	4.4g
saturated fat	0.8g
cholesterol	2mg
dietary fiber	8g
carbohydrate	22g
protein	8g
sodium	531mg

good source of: fiber, folate, thiamin, vitamin C

2 teaspoons oil
1 cup chopped green bell pepper
1 teaspoon minced garlic
1 can (19 ounces) black beans, rinsed and drained
1½ cups chicken broth
1 teaspoon coriander
1 teaspoon cumin
¼ cup plain fat-free yogurt

1 In a large nonstick saucepan, heat the oil over medium heat. Add the bell pepper and garlic, and cook, stirring occasionally, until the pepper is tender, about 5 minutes.

2 Stir in the beans, broth, coriander, and cumin, and bring to a boil. Reduce to a simmer, cover, and cook for 5 minutes to blend the flavors.

3 Transfer half the soup to a food processor. Puree and stir back into the soup. Serve the soup topped with the yogurt. ***Makes 4 servings***

Cream of Pumpkin Soup

Parmesan, pumpkin, and sage provide an interesting interplay of salty, sweet, and savory flavors in this rich-tasting soup.

per serving	
calories	168
total fat	4.4g
saturated fat	1.6g
cholesterol	8mg
dietary fiber	5g
carbohydrate	21g
protein	12g
sodium	668mg

good source of: beta carotene, calcium, fiber, riboflavin, vitamin D

2 teaspoons olive oil
½ cup chopped onion
1 teaspoon minced garlic
1 can (15 ounces) unsweetened pumpkin puree
1 can (12 ounces) evaporated fat-free milk
¾ teaspoon salt
½ teaspoon rubbed sage
½ teaspoon pepper
¼ cup grated Parmesan cheese

1 In a large nonstick saucepan, heat the oil over medium heat. Add the onion and garlic, and cook, stirring occasionally, until the onion is tender, about 7 minutes.

2 Add the pumpkin puree, evaporated milk, salt, sage, and pepper, and bring to a boil. Reduce to a simmer, cover, and cook for 5 minutes to blend the flavors. Stir in the Parmesan and serve. ***Makes 4 servings***

Pasta with Creamy Pumpkin Sauce Cook 10 ounces of ziti pasta according to package directions. Reduce the amount of evaporated milk in the soup to ¾ cup. Toss the sauce with the cooked pasta.

Crockpot cooking

Two principal compo-
nents of many West
African dishes are winter
squash and peanuts
(called ground nuts in
Africa). Here they are combined with turkey sausage,
rice, and black-eyed peas
in a delicious slow-cooked
soup. The soup will be perfectly cooked after 4 hours
but can go as long as 8.

West African Turkey & Squash Soup

2 cups frozen butternut squash cubes
1½ cups frozen black-eyed peas
½ cup brown rice
1 can (4 ounces) chopped mild green chilies, drained
2 tablespoons reduced-fat creamy peanut butter
4 teaspoons minced garlic
½ teaspoon oregano
½ teaspoon salt
3¼ cups water
½ pound sweet or hot Italian-style turkey sausages

1 In a 4- or 6-quart electric slow cooker, combine the butternut squash, black-eyed peas, rice, chilies, peanut butter, garlic, oregano, and salt.

2 Stir in the water and turkey sausages. Cover and cook on low for 4 to 8 hours or until the rice is tender and the sausages are cooked through. At serving time, remove the sausages, slice them, and return them to the pot. *Makes 4 servings*

PER SERVING 344 calories, 9.6g total fat (2.4g saturated), 43mg cholesterol, 9g dietary fiber, 46g carbohydrate, 21g protein, 917mg sodium
Good source of: beta carotene, fiber, folate, potassium, thiamin, vitamin C, zinc

F.Y.I.

For a modest number of calories and fat grams, this apparently unassuming soup has a wealth of healthful nutrients. The bulk of the B vitamins, including the folate, come from the asparagus, but the onions and potatoes make a contribution as well. The minerals—calcium, magnesium, potassium, and selenium—come primarily from the milk, with the potatoes and asparagus helping out. But, clearly, the asparagus is the nutritional star here.

Asparagus-Potato Soup

Mashed potato flakes make an almost instant cream soup with good potato flavor. If you have fresh dill on hand, you can use as much as ¼ cup chopped in place of the dried dillweed.

>   2 teaspoons olive oil
>   ½ cup chopped onion
>   2 teaspoons minced garlic
>   ¾ cup instant mashed potato flakes
>   ½ teaspoon dillweed
>   ¾ teaspoon salt
>   ½ teaspoon pepper
>   3 cups fat-free milk
>   1 package (10 ounces) frozen asparagus spears, thawed
>   and cut into 2-inch lengths

1 In a large nonstick saucepan, heat the oil over medium heat. Add the onion and garlic, and cook, stirring occasionally, until the onion is tender, about 7 minutes.

2 Stir in the potato flakes, dillweed, salt, pepper, and milk, stirring until smooth.

3 Bring to a simmer over medium heat. Reduce the heat to low and add the asparagus. Cook until the asparagus are tender, about 4 minutes. ***Makes 4 servings***

Mushroom-Potato Soup Substitute tarragon for the dill. Substitute 10 ounces of sliced cremini mushrooms for the asparagus, and cook them as directed in step 3.

Three-Pepper Gazpacho

per serving	
calories	113
total fat	3.7g
saturated fat	0.5g
cholesterol	0mg
dietary fiber	4g
carbohydrate	17g
protein	3g
sodium	792mg

good source of: beta carotene, fiber, potassium, vitamin B6, vitamin C

The three peppers in question are green bell pepper, roasted red pepper, and spicy jalapeño pepper. If you are using frozen chopped bell pepper and onion for this soup, you don't have to thaw them first, because gazpacho is intended to be eaten chilled. Although you could use a regular cucumber for the soup, kirby cukes have the advantage of a thin, unwaxed skin that you don't have to peel.

1 can (14½ ounces) stewed tomatoes
1 cup chopped onion
1 cup chopped green bell pepper
1 cup jarred roasted red peppers, rinsed and drained
1 pickled jalapeño pepper
2 kirby cucumbers, cut into large chunks
2 teaspoons minced garlic
3 tablespoons red wine vinegar
1 tablespoon olive oil
¾ teaspoon salt
¼ cup fresh basil leaves
¼ cup plain fat-free yogurt

1 In a blender or food processor, combine the stewed tomatoes, onion, green bell pepper, roasted red peppers, jalapeño, cucumbers, garlic, vinegar, oil, salt, and basil. Process until not quite smooth. Refrigerate several hours or until very cold.

2 Serve topped with a dollop of yogurt. *Makes 4 servings*

Curried Salmon Salad on Whole-Grain Toast

Although the fats in salmon are beneficial, it is still a high-fat food. So making a salad with salmon presents a challenge. The solution is fat-free sour cream jazzed up with lemon juice, curry powder, and sharp mustard.

> ⅓ cup fat-free sour cream
> ¼ cup chopped onion
> 3 tablespoons pickle relish
> 1 tablespoon lemon juice
> 1½ teaspoons curry powder
> ½ teaspoon Dijon mustard
> 1 can (14¾ ounces) pink salmon
> 8 slices whole-grain bread, toasted
> 1 cup cilantro leaves

1 In a large bowl, stir together the sour cream, onion, pickle relish, lemon juice, curry powder, and mustard. Add the salmon and stir to combine.

2 Make sandwiches with a layer of cilantro leaves on top of the salmon salad. *Makes 4 servings*

Curried Tuna Salad Sandwich Use plain low-fat yogurt instead of sour cream and substitute mango chutney for the pickle relish. Instead of salmon, use 2 cans (6 ounces each) of water-packed tuna.

F.Y.I.

While the sour cream provides a small amount of calcium, the majority of the bone-nourishing mineral in this salad comes from the canned salmon. The tiny bones in canned salmon are softened and delicate, making them entirely edible and nutritious. The average amount of calcium in ½ cup of canned salmon (with the bones) is 290 milligrams—only 10 milligrams less than the amount in 1 cup of milk.

Grilled Shrimp with Pineapple Salsa

per serving	
calories	224
total fat	3.2g
saturated fat	0.5g
cholesterol	135mg
dietary fiber	3g
carbohydrate	33g
protein	16g
sodium	585mg

good source of: selenium, vitamin B$_{12}$, vitamin C, vitamin D

As a change from the shrimp, try this pineapple salsa (step 1) with simple broiled or baked fish, such as Indian-Style Baked Cod (*page 44*), Simple Broiled Tuna Steak (*page 48*), or Broiled Chili-Rubbed Salmon (*page 46*).

3 tablespoons ketchup
3 tablespoons plus ¼ cup frozen pineapple juice
　　concentrate, thawed
2 tablespoons lime juice
1 teaspoon cumin
½ teaspoon salt
2 cups pineapple chunks
¼ cup chopped onion
2 teaspoons olive oil
1 pound large shrimp, shelled and deveined

1 In a large bowl, whisk together the ketchup, 3 tablespoons of the pineapple juice concentrate, the lime juice, ½ teaspoon of the cumin, and ¼ teaspoon of the salt. Add the pineapple and onion, tossing well to combine. Refrigerate until serving time.

2 In a large bowl, whisk together the remaining ½ teaspoon cumin, remaining ¼ teaspoon salt, the remaining ¼ cup pineapple juice concentrate, and oil. Add the shrimp and toss to coat well.

3 Spray a grill topper or broiler pan with nonstick cooking spray. Preheat the grill or broiler. Broil or grill the shrimp 4 to 6 inches from the heat until opaque throughout, 1½ to 2 minutes per side. Serve with the pineapple salsa.
Makes 4 servings

Asian-Style Broiled Swordfish

The marinade for the swordfish also works well with tuna steaks, salmon, snapper, grouper, and any number of flavorful firm-fleshed fish.

> ¼ cup chili sauce
> 2 tablespoons balsamic vinegar
> 2 teaspoons light brown sugar
> 2 teaspoons dark sesame oil
> ½ teaspoon ground ginger
> ¼ teaspoon salt
> 4 swordfish steaks (6 ounces each)

1 In a shallow bowl, combine the chili sauce, vinegar, brown sugar, sesame oil, ginger, and salt. Add the swordfish and marinate in the refrigerator for at least 1 hour, turning the fish over midway.

2 Preheat the broiler. Spray a broiler pan with nonstick cooking spray. Lift the fish from the marinade and place on the broiler pan. Spoon any remaining marinade over the fish. Broil 4 to 6 inches from the heat for 4 to 6 minutes, or until the fish just flakes when tested with a fork. ***Makes 4 servings***

Asian-Style Swordfish Salad Make a double batch of marinade (step 1) and transfer half of it to a large bowl to serve as salad dressing. Marinate the swordfish in the remaining marinade (in the refrigerator) and broil as directed. At serving time, to the bowl of reserved salad dressing, add 8 cups mixed salad greens, 1 cup mandarin orange or grapefruit sections, and 1 can (8 ounces) drained sliced water chestnuts. Toss together. Serve the broiled swordfish on a bed of the salad.

ON THE *Menu*

Though the percentage of calories from saturated fat is low (7%), to balance out the total fat that comes with this simple broiled swordfish, keep the rest of the meal relatively low-fat. If you serve brown rice and steamed sugar snap peas on the side, you'll bring the percentage of calories from fat for the dinner down to about 19% (and the saturated fat to 4%). Then you can even treat yourself to a gooey dessert. Try Sweet Cherry Sundaes (*page 127*).

Fresh Tuna & Potato Salad

If you'd prefer, simply use canned tuna and flake it over the potato salad. Skinless chicken breast, grilled flank steak, or shrimp would also work well.

per serving	
calories	361
total fat	5.7g
saturated fat	1.3g
cholesterol	35mg
dietary fiber	6g
carbohydrate	52g
protein	28g
sodium	698mg

good source of: folate, magnesium, niacin, omega-3 fatty acids, potassium, riboflavin, selenium, thiamin, vitamin B_{12}, vitamin B_6, vitamin C, vitamin D

1½ pounds small red or white potatoes, unpeeled
¾ pound tuna steaks
¾ teaspoon salt
⅓ cup distilled white vinegar
2 tablespoons Dijon mustard
1 teaspoon minced garlic
1 teaspoon dillweed
½ teaspoon pepper
1 cup frozen corn kernels, thawed
6 cups mixed salad greens

1 In a large pot of boiling water, cook the potatoes until fork-tender, about 20 minutes. Drain the potatoes and when cool enough to handle, thickly slice them.

2 Meanwhile, preheat the broiler. Place the tuna on a broiler pan. Sprinkle ¼ teaspoon of the salt over the tuna and broil 4 to 6 inches from the heat until medium-rare (still slightly pink in the center), about 5 minutes. Let cool to room temperature.

3 In a large bowl, combine the remaining ½ teaspoon salt, the vinegar, mustard, garlic, dillweed, and pepper. Add the sliced potatoes and corn to the bowl and toss to combine.

4 Place the salad greens on a large platter. Top with the potato salad. Thinly slice the tuna and place on top of the potato salad. ***Makes 4 servings***

Scallops, Mushrooms & Peas au Gratin

per serving	
calories	288
total fat	4.1g
saturated fat	1.7g
cholesterol	45mg
dietary fiber	4g
carbohydrate	32g
protein	31g
sodium	902mg

good source of:
riboflavin, selenium, thiamin, vitamin B_{12}

Small, tender bay scallops are perfect for this creamy gratin, but they are seasonal. So if bay scallops are not available, make the gratin with small shrimp, shelled and deveined.

⅓ cup water
8 ounces sliced mushrooms
2 cups low-fat (1%) milk
¼ cup flour
1 cup frozen peas, thawed
¾ teaspoon salt
¼ teaspoon cayenne pepper
1 pound bay scallops
½ cup plain dried breadcrumbs
2 tablespoons grated Parmesan cheese

1 In a large nonstick skillet, combine the water and mushrooms, and bring to a boil over medium heat. Cook, stirring frequently, until the mushrooms are tender and the liquid has evaporated, about 5 minutes. Set aside.

2 In a medium saucepan, whisk the milk into the flour. Bring to a simmer over medium heat and cook, stirring frequently, until the sauce is the consistency of heavy cream, about 5 minutes. Stir in the mushrooms, peas, salt, and cayenne.

3 Place the scallops in a shallow 7 x 11-inch broilerproof dish. Pour the mushroom-pea sauce over the scallops.

4 In a small bowl, combine the breadcrumbs and Parmesan. Scatter the mixture over the scallops and broil for 2 minutes, or until the scallops are just opaque and the sauce is piping hot. *Makes 4 servings*

ON THE *Menu*

To round out the meal, and make the percentage of calories from fat lower, serve the swordfish with parslied rice, steamed green beans, and roasted red peppers. For dessert, offer Baked Bananas (*page 129*).

Broiled Salmon with Spicy Corn Salad

The corn salad that tops this broiled salmon couldn't be simpler. But if you're in the mood for something a little more elaborate, skip the corn salad and make the Pineapple Salsa that goes with the grilled shrimp on page 37 instead.

    1½ cups frozen corn kernels, thawed
    ½ cup bottled medium salsa
    ½ teaspoon cumin
    ½ teaspoon coriander
    ¼ teaspoon salt
    4 skinless salmon fillets (5 ounces each)

1 Preheat the broiler. In a medium bowl, combine the corn, salsa, cumin, and coriander.

2 Sprinkle the salt over the salmon. Place the salmon on a broiler pan and broil 4 to 6 inches from the heat until the salmon just flakes when tested with a fork. Serve the salmon with the corn salad spooned on top. *Makes 4 servings*

Broiled Salmon with Curried Corn Salad In step 1, omit the cumin and coriander and use 1½ teaspoons of curry powder. Stir 2 tablespoons mango chutney into the corn salad.

Fish Florentine with Orange Sauce

The term "florentine" in a recipe name implies that the food will be served on a bed of spinach and topped with either grated cheese or a cheese sauce.

<table>
<tr><td colspan="2">per serving</td></tr>
<tr><td>calories</td><td>231</td></tr>
<tr><td>total fat</td><td>4.3g</td></tr>
<tr><td>saturated fat</td><td>0.8g</td></tr>
<tr><td>cholesterol</td><td>68mg</td></tr>
<tr><td>dietary fiber</td><td>3g</td></tr>
<tr><td>carbohydrate</td><td>19g</td></tr>
<tr><td>protein</td><td>30g</td></tr>
<tr><td>sodium</td><td>617mg</td></tr>
</table>

good source of: beta carotene, folate, magnesium, niacin, potassium, selenium, vitamin B_{12}, vitamin B_6, vitamin C, vitamin E

2 teaspoons olive oil
1 teaspoon minced garlic
1 package (16 ounces) frozen chopped spinach, thawed and drained
⅔ cup orange juice
⅓ cup raisins
¾ teaspoon salt
¼ teaspoon pepper
¼ teaspoon oregano
4 tilapia fillets (5 ounces each)
3 tablespoons grated Parmesan cheese

1 In a large nonstick skillet, heat the oil over low heat. Add the garlic and cook until tender, about 1 minute. Add the spinach, orange juice, raisins, ½ teaspoon of the salt, the pepper, and oregano, and bring to a boil.

2 Place the fish on top of the spinach and sprinkle with the remaining ¼ teaspoon salt and the Parmesan. Cover and cook until the fish just flakes when tested with a fork and the spinach is heated through, about 5 minutes. *Makes 4 servings*

Chicken Florentine Use 4 skinless, boneless chicken breast halves (5 ounces each) instead of the fish. In step 1, add ¼ cup water and substitute rosemary for the oregano. In step 2, cook the chicken for 15 minutes.

F.Y.I.

This light but satisfying salad provides 1.81 mcg of vitamin B_{12} with a small amount coming from the yogurt, but the lion's share coming from the shrimp. Vitamin B_{12} is required to manufacture blood cells and to maintain the integrity of nervous and gastrointestinal systems. Meat, fish, dairy products, and fortified cereals are all rich sources of the vitamin. The RDA for vitamin B_{12} is 2.4 mcg, which for most adults can be obtained through food. However, vitamin B_{12} deficiency may still occur in 10% to 30% of older people because of a diminished ability to absorb B_{12} from food. Therefore, healthcare professionals may advise that adults over the age of 50 get their RDA for vitamin B_{12} from a supplement.

Shrimp Louis

This light and easy-to-prepare shrimp salad is based on Crab Louis, a classic dish variously attributed to a chef in Seattle or one of two chefs in San Francisco. In addition to having multiple inventors, the dish also has multiple versions, though all are cold salads that invariably include a creamy dressing made with chili sauce.

⅓ cup plain fat-free yogurt
2 tablespoons chili sauce
1 teaspoon capers
½ teaspoon tarragon
¼ teaspoon pepper
1 pound cooked, shelled shrimp
1 cup small cherry or grape tomatoes
4 cups mixed salad greens
¼ cup storebought guacamole

1 In a large bowl, stir together the yogurt, chili sauce, capers, tarragon, and pepper.

2 Add the shrimp and tomatoes to the bowl and toss to coat.

3 Arrange the mixed greens on 4 serving plates and spoon the shrimp mixture on top. Place a dollop of guacamole on top. *Makes 4 servings*

Indian-Style Baked Cod

per serving	
calories	115
total fat	1.8g
saturated fat	0.8g
cholesterol	41mg
dietary fiber	0g
carbohydrate	5g
protein	19g
sodium	388mg

good source of: selenium, vitamin B_{12}

Serve this dish with basmati or jasmati rice and a small dish of mango chutney. The marinade for this baked cod would work equally well with grouper or snapper.

1 cup plain low-fat yogurt
1½ teaspoons cumin
¾ teaspoon coriander
½ teaspoon ground ginger
½ teaspoon salt
½ teaspoon pepper
4 cod steaks (6 ounces each)

1 In a 7 x 11-inch baking dish, stir together the yogurt, cumin, coriander, ginger, salt, and pepper. Add the cod and turn to coat with the spiced yogurt mixture.

2 Refrigerate for at least 1 hour or up to 4 hours. Bring to room temperature before baking.

3 Preheat the oven to 450°F. Bake for 15 minutes, or until the fish just flakes when tested with a fork. Lift the fish from the cooking mixture to serve. Remove any skin before eating. ***Makes 4 servings***

Baked Indian-Style Chicken Substitute 4 skinless, boneless chicken breast halves (5 ounces each) for the cod. Bake for 15 to 20 minutes, or until the chicken is cooked through.

F.Y.I.

Lemon pepper is a blend of black pepper, citric acid, lemon oil, and garlic. Depending on the manufacturer, it can also contain salt and other spices. It's a good way to get some of the flavor of lemon zest without having to grate fresh lemon peel.

Curry-Broiled Swordfish with Honey Sauce

Tart lemon juice balances the sweetness of the honey in the curry-flavored sauce for this broiled swordfish. Instead of swordfish, you could use another sturdy fish, such as cod or halibut.

> 1½ teaspoons curry powder
> 1 teaspoon cumin
> ¾ teaspoon salt
> ¾ teaspoon lemon-pepper
> 4 swordfish steaks (6 ounces each)
> ⅓ cup lemon juice
> ⅓ cup honey
> ½ cup jarred roasted red peppers, diced (optional)

1 Preheat the broiler. In a small bowl, combine the curry powder, cumin, salt, and lemon-pepper. Measure out 2 teaspoons of the spice mixture and rub it into the swordfish.

2 Place the swordfish on a broiler pan and broil 4 to 6 inches from the heat for 3 minutes per side, or until it just flakes when tested with a fork.

3 Add the lemon juice, honey, and roasted red pepper (if using) to the spice mixture remaining in the bowl. Serve the hot fish with the sauce spooned on top. *Makes 4 servings*

Mexican-Style Broiled Swordfish In step 1, omit the curry powder and add 2 teaspoons coriander and ½ teaspoon oregano to the spice mixture. In step 3, use lime juice instead of lemon juice in the sauce.

Broiled Chili-Rubbed Salmon

If you like this easy chili rub for salmon, make up a big batch of it to keep on hand for flavoring chicken or turkey breast, or pork tenderloin. To make enough spice for about 5 pounds of fish, poultry, or meat, combine 3 tablespoons chili powder, 1 tablespoon each of cumin and salt, and 2 teaspoons sugar.

> 1 tablespoon mild chili powder
> ¾ teaspoon cumin
> ¾ teaspoon salt
> ½ teaspoon sugar
> 4 skinless salmon fillets (5 ounces each)

1 Preheat the broiler. In a small bowl, combine the chili powder, cumin, salt, and sugar. Rub the mixture into both sides of the salmon.

2 Place the salmon on a broiler pan and broil 4 to 6 inches from the heat without turning, until the fish just flakes when tested with a fork, about 6 minutes. ***Makes 4 servings***

Chili-Orange Pork Make the spice mixture in step 1 and rub it into a 1- to 1¼-pound pork tenderloin. In a small bowl, stir together 2 tablespoons orange all-fruit spread and 1 tablespoon lemon juice. Roast the pork at 425°F for 25 minutes. Brush it with the orange mixture and roast 10 to 15 minutes longer, or until cooked through but still juicy.

ON THE *Menu*

Serve the salmon with side dishes of quick-cooking barley and steamed baby spinach. If you're feeling ambitious, make a spicy accompaniment to go with the salmon. Try Spicy Corn Salad (*page 41*), Tomato-Horseradish Topping (*page 52*), or Pineapple Salsa (*page 37*). For dessert, have chilled sliced oranges tossed with toasted slivered almonds.

Tomato-Braised Scallops

These scallops are gently braised in a basil-tomato sauce underscored by the sweetness of beta carotene-rich carrot juice. Serve the scallops over rice or freshly cooked pasta (orzo would be good), or with chunks of crusty peasant bread for mopping up the sauce.

per serving	
calories	190
total fat	3.5g
saturated fat	0.5g
cholesterol	37mg
dietary fiber	4g
carbohydrate	17g
protein	23g
sodium	580mg

good source of:
beta carotene, selenium, vitamin B_{12}

2 teaspoons olive oil
2 teaspoons minced garlic
1 cup canned crushed tomatoes
¾ cup carrot juice
2 tablespoons chopped basil
½ teaspoon salt
1 pound sea scallops
1½ cups frozen peas (no need to thaw)

1 In a large nonstick skillet, heat the oil over low heat. Add the garlic and cook until tender, about 1 minute.

2 Add the tomatoes, carrot juice, basil, and salt, and bring to a boil. Boil for 2 minutes to blend the flavors.

3 Reduce to a simmer and add the scallops and peas. Cover and cook until the scallops are just opaque and the peas are heated through, about 3 minutes. *Makes 4 servings*

KITCHENtip

Sea scallops can be quite large (sometimes close to 2 inches across). If you have a fish store or supermarket seafood department that will indulge you, ask them to give you the smallest scallops possible. This way you get more mileage out of the pound that you are buying.

ON THE *Menu*

Serve the tuna with Carrot & Raisin Couscous (*page 114*) and steamed asparagus. Follow with an arugula and grape tomato salad in a low-fat vinaigrette. For dessert, offer Orange-Broiled Angel Food Cake with Mocha Sauce (*page 128*).

Simple Broiled Tuna Steak

This marinade works equally well with bluefish, salmon, or mackerel. For a real change of pace, try the marinade on skinless, boneless chicken breasts.

> ¼ cup reduced-sodium soy sauce
> 2 tablespoons light brown sugar
> 1 teaspoon minced ginger
> 1 teaspoon minced garlic
> 2 teaspoons lemon juice
> 2 tuna steaks (10 ounces each)

1 In a shallow bowl, stir together the soy sauce, brown sugar, ginger, garlic, and lemon juice. Place the tuna in the marinade and refrigerate for 1 hour, turning the tuna over midway.

2 Preheat the broiler. Lift the tuna from the marinade and place on a broiler pan. Spoon half the marinade over the tuna. Broil the tuna 4 to 6 inches from the heat for 3 minutes. Pour the remaining marinade over the tuna and broil until the tuna is medium-rare (cooked through but still slightly pink in the center), about 2 minutes.

3 Cut the tuna steaks in half for a total of 4 serving pieces. ***Makes 4 servings***

Parmesan-Crusted Tilapia

Though the firm, meaty texture of tilapia is perfect here, you could also use a mild fish such as flounder or sole.

2 tablespoons light mayonnaise
1 tablespoon reduced-fat sour cream
2 teaspoons coarse-grained Dijon mustard
1/2 teaspoon salt
1/4 teaspoon pepper
4 skinless tilapia fillets (about 6 ounces each)
3 tablespoons grated Parmesan cheese
1/4 cup plain dried breadcrumbs

1 Preheat the broiler. Spray a jelly-roll pan or baking sheet with nonstick cooking spray.

2 In a small bowl, stir together the mayonnaise, sour cream, mustard, salt, and pepper.

3 Arrange the tilapia in a single layer on the pan. Spread the mayonnaise mixture evenly over the fish and sprinkle evenly with the Parmesan.

4 Broil the fish 4 to 6 inches from the heat for 3 minutes. Sprinkle the breadcrumbs over the fish and broil for 1 minute, or until the the topping is golden brown and the fish just flakes when tested with a fork. ***Makes 4 servings***

Spicy Parmesan-Crusted Snapper In step 2, omit the mustard and add 1 tablespoon horseradish, and use cayenne pepper instead of black pepper. Substitute red snapper fillets for the tilapia.

F.Y.I.

Sometimes called sunshine snapper or St. Peter's fish, tilapia is an important farm-raised fish. Once largely imported, it is now being farmed in this country and is widely available in supermarkets. Tilapia has firm flesh and a mild, meaty taste that should please anyone not fond of fishy-tasting fish.

Soy-Ginger Salmon

per serving	
calories	237
total fat	10g
saturated fat	1.6g
cholesterol	81mg
dietary fiber	0g
carbohydrate	5g
protein	29g
sodium	465mg

good source of: niacin, omega-3 fatty acids, potassium, riboflavin, selenium, thiamin, vitamin B$_{12}$, vitamin B$_6$, vitamin D

ON THE *Menu*

Serve this simple broiled salmon with Smashed Potato Salad (*page 110*) and steamed baby carrots. For dessert, have Fresh Blueberry Granola Crisp (*page 132*).

If you happen to have bottled ginger juice on hand (*see page 65 for more information on ginger juice*), you could use it instead of the fresh ginger. Use 1 teaspoon of ginger juice in place of the minced ginger.

> 4 salmon steaks (6 ounces each)
> 3 tablespoons reduced-sodium soy sauce
> 1 tablespoon light brown sugar
> 1 teaspoon dark sesame oil
> 2 teaspoons minced fresh ginger
> ½ teaspoon dried orange peel

1 Preheat the broiler. Place the salmon on a broiler pan.

2 In a shallow bowl, stir together the soy sauce, brown sugar, sesame oil, ginger, and orange peel.

3 Brush the mixture over the top of the salmon. Broil 4 to 6 inches from the heat until the salmon just flakes when tested with a fork, about 6 minutes. *Makes 4 servings*

Soy-Ginger Salmon Salad Make a double batch of the soy-ginger baste (step 2) and transfer half of it to a serving bowl to serve as a salad dressing. Baste and cook the salmon as directed. To the dressing, add 2 cups cooked rice, 1 cup green peas, and 1 cup shredded carrots. Cut the broiled salmon into bite-size pieces, add to the salad, and toss gently to combine.

Tuna, Corn & Cheddar Frittata

Flaking canned tuna is merely a method of breaking up the tight layers of cooked fish. This allows the tuna to combine evenly with the other frittata ingredients. If you can't find Mexican corn, just use regular canned corn.

2 teaspoons olive oil
½ cup chopped onion
1½ cups canned Mexican corn (corn & peppers), drained
1 can (3 ounces) water-packed tuna, drained and flaked
1 cup egg substitute
¼ teaspoon salt
½ cup shredded reduced-fat Cheddar cheese

1 In a large nonstick skillet, heat 1 teaspoon of the oil over low heat. Add the onion and cook until tender, about 7 minutes.

2 Transfer the onion to a large bowl and stir in the corn and tuna. Add the egg substitute, salt, and ¼ cup of the Cheddar, and stir to combine.

3 Add the remaining 1 teaspoon oil to the skillet and heat over low heat. Pour the egg mixture into the pan and cook, without stirring, until set, about 15 minutes.

4 Scatter the remaining ¼ cup of Cheddar over the frittata. Cover and cook until the cheese has melted, about 3 minutes. *Makes 4 servings*

KITCHEN *tip*

Ordinarily when we create a recipe with storebought egg substitute, we offer the alternative of using egg whites. But for this frittata, we would propose adding at least 1 whole egg for a little bit of flavor with minimal fat. So for the 1 cup of egg substitute called for, use 6 egg whites and 1 whole egg instead.

Broiled Bluefish with Tomato-Horseradish Topping

Bluefish is a wonderfully meaty and flavorful fish, but it can have a fishy flavor (especially in the darker portions of the fillet) when it's not at its freshest. If you are not sure that your market's bluefish is absolutely fresh, use another, milder fish, such as tilapia, instead.

2 tablespoons fat-free sour cream
2 tablespoons ketchup
1 tablespoon light mayonnaise
2 teaspoons drained white horseradish
4 bluefish fillets (5 ounces each)
4 teaspoons lemon juice
½ teaspoon salt
¼ teaspoon pepper
¼ cup plain dried breadcrumbs

1 Preheat the broiler. In a small bowl, combine the sour cream, ketchup, mayonnaise, and horseradish.

2 Place the fish on a broiler pan. Drizzle the fillets with the lemon juice and sprinkle with the salt and pepper. Broil 4 to 6 inches from the heat for 5 minutes.

3 Spread the horseradish mixture over the fish. Sprinkle the breadcrumbs over the top. Broil the fish for 2 minutes, or until the topping is lightly browned and the fish just flakes when tested with a fork. *Makes 4 servings*

per serving	
calories	235
total fat	7.8g
saturated fat	1.5g
cholesterol	87mg
dietary fiber	0g
carbohydrate	9g
protein	30g
sodium	571mg

good source of: niacin, omega-3 fatty acids, selenium, vitamin B_{12}, vitamin B_6

F.Y.I.

Although all bell peppers provide fiber and vitamin B_6, there are some nutritional differences that depend on the color of the pepper. For example, yellow and red bell peppers have more than twice the amount of vitamin C in green peppers. And red peppers contain eleven times more beta carotene than green peppers.

Salmon-Pasta Salad with Creamy Lemon Dressing

Pureeing roasted yellow peppers with some yogurt, mayonnaise, and lemon juice makes a creamy lemon-colored dressing for canned salmon, kidney beans, and pasta.

½ cup jarred roasted yellow peppers, rinsed and drained
½ cup plain fat-free yogurt
2 tablespoons light mayonnaise
2 tablespoons lemon juice
¼ teaspoon salt
1 can (14¾ ounces) sockeye salmon
1 cup canned kidney beans, rinsed and drained
8 ounces penne pasta

1 In a food processor, combine the peppers, yogurt, mayonnaise, lemon juice, and salt, and puree. Transfer the dressing to a large bowl. Add the salmon and beans, and toss to combine.

2 Meanwhile, in a large pot of boiling water, cook the penne according to package directions. Drain.

3 Add the drained pasta to the bowl and toss to combine. Serve at room temperature or chilled. *Makes 4 servings*

Tuna-Pasta Salad with Pepper Pesto In the dressing, step 1, substitute roasted red peppers for the yellow and decrease the amount of mayonnaise to 1 tablespoon. Add 1 tablespoon storebought pesto to the dressing before pureeing. Use 2 cans (6 ounces each) of water-packed tuna instead of salmon, and cannellini beans instead of the kidney beans. Add ⅓ cup chopped onion.

On the *Menu*

If you have a barbecue grill, grill the fish outdoors. Use some extra chili sauce to brush on portobello mushrooms and grill them along with the fish. For a salad, toss shredded carrots with fat-free ranch dressing. Offer Tropical Fruit Compote (*page 135*) for dessert.

Chili-Barbecued Red Snapper

You can skip the corn relish for this recipe if you'd like, and serve jarred piccalilli instead.

> ½ cup chili sauce
> ¼ cup red wine vinegar
> 2 tablespoons honey
> 4 red snapper fillets (6 ounces each)
> 2 cups frozen corn kernels, thawed
> ½ cup jarred roasted red peppers, drained and diced

1 Preheat the broiler. In a medium bowl, stir together the chili sauce, vinegar, and honey. Place the snapper, skin-side down, on a broiler pan and spoon half the chili sauce mixture over the fish.

2 Add the corn and roasted red peppers to the chili sauce mixture remaining in the bowl.

3 Broil the snapper 4 to 6 inches from the heat for 7 minutes, or until it just flakes when tested with a fork. Serve the snapper with the corn relish spooned on top. ***Makes 4 servings***

Chili-Barbecued Turkey Burgers Use 4 packaged lean turkey burgers (4 ounces each) instead of the snapper fillets. Baste and broil as directed, but let the burgers cook 5 to 7 minutes to be sure they are cooked through. Serve the burgers on whole-grain rolls with romaine lettuce. Serve the corn salad on the side or as a sandwich topping.

Crockpot cooking

White Chili

1½ cups (9 ounces) dried white beans, such as
   cannellini or Great Northern, rinsed and picked over
3 cups water
1½ pounds pork, cut for stir-fry
1 pound small white potatoes
1 cup chopped onion
1 tablespoon minced garlic
1 can (11 ounces) white shoepeg corn, drained
2 tablespoons jalapeño pepper sauce
¾ teaspoon oregano
¾ teaspoon coriander
1½ teaspoons salt
2 tablespoons flour

1 In a large bowl, combine the beans and water to cover by several inches. Let soak overnight. Drain.

2 In a 6-quart electric slow cooker, combine the drained beans and 2 cups of the water, and cook on high heat for 1 hour.

3 Add the pork, potatoes, onion, garlic, corn, jalapeño pepper sauce, oregano, coriander, and salt.

4 Cover and cook on low heat until the beans, pork, and potatoes are tender, about 8 hours.

5 In a small bowl, stir the remaining 1 cup of water into the flour until smooth. Stir the flour mixture into the slow cooker and cook until the sauce is thickened, about 15 minutes. ***Makes 8 servings***

PER SERVING **414 calories, 9.8g total fat (3.5g saturated), 52mg cholesterol, 12g dietary fiber, 53g carbohydrate, 29g protein, 795mg sodium**
Good source of: **fiber, folate, niacin, potassium, selenium, thiamin, vitamin B₆, zinc**

White beans, white corn, pork ("the other white meat"), and white potatoes give this slow-cooked chili an unexpected color, but a hearty flavor. If you like, serve the chili with shredded reduced-fat Monterey jack cheese and plain fat-free yogurt (just to keep the same color theme going). If you're making this chili in warm weather, put the bowl of beans in the refrigerator to soak overnight. If you don't want to start with dried beans, substitute 3¾ cups canned beans (from about two 19-ounce cans) and omit steps 1 and 2.

ON THE *Menu*

To take full advantage of the delicious sauce for these cutlets (and to get a better balance of fat to calories), serve the pork with rice. As a side dish, try a steamed green vegetable, such as broccoli rabe, Italian green beans, or spinach.

Sautéed Pork Cutlets with Pineapple-Cherry Sauce

Making a pan sauce with fruit juice is a quick and healthful way to dress up sautéed pork cutlets. The cornstarch gives the sauce a rich, smooth texture.

4 well-trimmed boneless pork loin chops (4 ounces each)
¼ teaspoon pepper
½ teaspoon salt
2 teaspoons olive oil
½ cup pineapple juice
½ cup chicken broth
2 teaspoons cornstarch
¼ cup dried cherries

1 Sprinkle the pork with the pepper and ¼ teaspoon of the salt. In a large nonstick skillet, heat the oil over medium heat. Add the pork to the pan and cook until golden brown, about 3 minutes per side. Transfer the pork to a plate.

2 In a small bowl or measuring cup, blend the pineapple juice, broth, and cornstarch. Add the remaining ¼ teaspoon salt and the pineapple juice mixture to the skillet and bring to a boil over medium heat, stirring to scrape up the browned bits from the bottom of the skillet.

3 Add the cherries and cook for 1 minute. Return the pork (and any juices that have collected on the plate) to the skillet and cook just until the pork is heated through, about 1 minute longer. ***Makes 4 servings***

per serving	
calories	194
total fat	4.3g
saturated fat	1.4g
cholesterol	74mg
dietary fiber	0g
carbohydrate	14g
protein	24g
sodium	496mg

good source of:
niacin, riboflavin, selenium, thiamin, vitamin B_{12}, vitamin B_6

ON THE *Menu*

For dinner, serve the slices of roast pork with mashed sweet potatoes and sliced tomatoes. Serve Boston lettuce with minced chives and fat-free Caesar dressing. For dessert, offer Cherry Clafouti (*page 134*). For lunch (assuming you have leftovers from dinner), make a sandwich with the sliced pork and lots of lettuce on whole-grain toast spread with a combination of fat-free mayonnaise and apricot jam.

Apricot-Glazed Roast Pork

If you like the apricot glaze for this pork, you might want to make a double or triple batch and keep it in the refrigerator for brushing on chicken breasts to be grilled.

¼ cup apricot jam
1 tablespoon ketchup
1 tablespoon Dijon mustard
2 teaspoons red wine vinegar
1 pound pork tenderloin
¾ teaspoon rubbed sage
½ teaspoon salt

1 Preheat the oven to 425°F. In a small bowl, combine the jam, ketchup, mustard, and vinegar.

2 Line a small roasting pan with foil (for easy cleanup). Place the pork in the pan and rub the sage and salt into the pork. Roast for 10 minutes.

3 Brush the pork with half of the jam mixture and roast for 10 minutes.

4 Brush with the remaining jam mixture and roast until the pork is cooked through but still juicy, about 10 minutes. Let stand for 5 minutes before thinly slicing. *Makes 4 servings*

Apricot-Glazed Chicken In step 2, omit the sage and use ½ teaspoon thyme and ¼ teaspoon rosemary to rub into 4 skinless, boneless chicken breast halves (5 ounces each). Bake for 5 minutes. Brush all of the apricot mixture on the chicken and bake for 7 to 10 minutes longer, or until cooked through.

Off-the-Shelf

One of the tricks to successful off-the-shelf cooking is knowing how to tweak a packaged product to make it not only better for your health but also more interesting. Using plain fat-free yogurt instead of milk in the corn muffin topping makes it tender and rich tasting, and a bit of added chili powder gives it a little kick.

Easy Tamale Pie

¼ cup water
2 teaspoons minced garlic
½ pound extra-lean ground beef
1 can (14½ ounces) crushed tomatoes
1 cup frozen corn kernels
2 teaspoons chili powder
½ teaspoon salt
2 tablespoons chopped green or black olives
1 box (8½ ounces) corn muffin mix
½ cup plain fat-free yogurt
2 large egg whites

1 Preheat the oven to 400°F. Spray a 9-inch pie plate with nonstick cooking spray.

2 In a large nonstick skillet, bring the water and garlic to a simmer over medium heat and cook until the garlic is tender, about 1 minute. Add the beef and cook until no longer pink, about 2 minutes.

3 Stir in the tomatoes, corn, 1 teaspoon of the chili powder, the salt, and olives, and simmer until the meat is cooked through and the mixture is flavorful, about 5 minutes.

4 In a large bowl, stir together the remaining 1 teaspoon chili powder, the corn muffin mix, yogurt, and egg whites until well combined. Spoon half the corn-muffin mixture into the pie plate. Top with the meat mixture and the remaining corn muffin mixture.

5 Place the pie plate on a baking sheet and bake until the top is set and golden brown, about 20 minutes. ***Makes 6 servings***

PER SERVING 299 calories, 9.2g total fat (2.7g saturated), 15mg cholesterol, 5g dietary fiber, 41g carbohydrate, 15g protein, 878mg sodium
Good source of: vitamin B_{12}

Beef & Barley Stew

Traditional stews use fattier cuts of beef like chuck, and the meat cooks along with the other stew ingredients. But when you use a lean cut of meat, you can't let it cook for that long or it will be dry and tough. Instead, we cook the meat very briefly in a skillet and then add it to the stew at the end so the beef stays juicy and tender.

2 cups chicken broth
1½ cups water
⅓ cup pearl barley
2 teaspoons minced garlic
½ teaspoon thyme
¼ teaspoon pepper
3 cups peeled baby carrots
1 cup chopped onion
2 teaspoons olive oil
¾ pound beef, cut for stir-fry
1 can (28 ounces) crushed tomatoes

1 In a large saucepan, combine the broth, water, barley, garlic, thyme, and pepper. Cover and bring to a boil over high heat. Reduce to low and simmer for 20 minutes.

2 Add the carrots and onion. Increase the heat to medium and bring to a boil. Reduce the heat to low, cover, and simmer, stirring occasionally, until the barley and carrots are tender, about 15 minutes.

3 Meanwhile, in a large nonstick skillet, heat the oil over high heat. Add the beef and sauté until browned, 3 to 4 minutes.

4 Add the tomatoes to the stew. Increase the heat to medium and bring to a boil. Cook, uncovered, for 5 minutes to blend the flavors. Stir in the beef and serve. *Makes 4 servings*

Chicken & Barley Stew In step 1, use tarragon instead of thyme. Use chicken cut for stir-fry instead of beef.

Wagon Wheels with Mexican Beef Sauce

per serving	
calories	442
total fat	9.5g
saturated fat	3.2g
cholesterol	21mg
dietary fiber	9g
carbohydrate	64g
protein	25g
sodium	644mg

good source of: fiber, folate, niacin, riboflavin, selenium, thiamin, vitamin B_{12}, vitamin C, zinc

Wagon-wheel pasta not only has eye appeal, but is an easy pasta to capture on the fork. It also has the bonus of catching the chunky sauce in its spokes, so every mouthful is rewarding.

8 ounces wagon-wheel pasta
2 teaspoons olive oil
½ cup chopped onion
1½ teaspoons minced garlic
6 ounces extra-lean ground beef
4 teaspoons chili powder
¼ teaspoon salt
1 can (14½ ounces) crushed tomatoes
1 can (15 ounces) black beans, rinsed and drained
1 tablespoon pickled jalapeño pepper slices
⅓ cup shredded reduced-fat sharp Cheddar cheese

1 In a large pot of boiling water, cook the pasta according to package directions. Drain and transfer to a serving bowl.

2 Meanwhile, in a large nonstick skillet, heat the oil over medium-high heat. Add the onion and garlic, and cook for 30 seconds.

3 Crumble in the ground beef. Sprinkle with the chili powder and salt, and cook, stirring occasionally, until the beef is no longer pink, about 5 minutes.

4 Add the tomatoes, black beans, and jalapeños, and bring to a boil over high heat. Reduce the heat to medium, cover, and cook for 5 minutes.

5 Add the beef sauce to the pasta. Sprinkle with the Cheddar and toss to mix. *Makes 4 servings*

Crockpot cooking

Irish Lamb & Vegetable Stew

2½ cups water
2 tablespoons flour
1 pound lean leg of lamb, cut for stew
1½ pounds small red potatoes
1½ cups frozen rutabaga chunks
1½ cups peeled baby carrots
1 cup chopped onion
1 tablespoon minced garlic
2 tablespoons tomato paste
1 teaspoon salt
¾ teaspoon thyme
1½ cups frozen peas

1 In a 4- to 6-quart electric slow cooker, stir the water into the flour until smooth. Add the lamb, potatoes, rutabaga, carrots, onion, garlic, tomato paste, salt, and thyme.

2 Cook on low until the meat and potatoes are tender, 6 to 8 hours. Add the peas and continue to cook until heated through, about 10 minutes. *Makes 6 servings*

PER SERVING 289 calories, 3.9g total fat (1.3g saturated), 48mg cholesterol, 7g dietary fiber, 42g carbohydrate, 22g protein, 554mg sodium
Good source of: beta carotene, niacin, potassium, riboflavin, selenium, thiamin, vitamin B$_{12}$, vitamin B$_6$, vitamin C, zinc

Pork Cutlets with Peanut-Lime Sauce

The tartness of lime juice balanced against the sweetness of brown sugar and the savory richness of peanut butter make a delicious sauce for broiled pork cutlets.

¼ cup lime juice
3 tablespoons brown sugar
½ teaspoon coriander
¼ teaspoon salt
2 tablespoons reduced-fat creamy peanut butter
1 tablespoon reduced-sodium soy sauce
½ teaspoon minced garlic
½ teaspoon minced ginger
4 well-trimmed boneless loin pork chops (4 ounces each)

1 In a small bowl, stir together 2 tablespoons of the lime juice, 2 tablespoons of the brown sugar, the coriander, and salt. Set the lime-brown sugar mixture aside to use as a baste for the pork.

2 In a food processor, combine the remaining 2 tablespoons lime juice, remaining 1 tablespoon brown sugar, the peanut butter, soy sauce, garlic, and ginger, and puree until smooth. Set the peanut-lime mixture aside to serve as a dipping sauce.

3 Preheat the broiler. Place the pork on a broiler pan and brush both sides with the reserved lime-brown sugar baste. Broil 4 to 6 inches from the heat for 5 minutes, or until the pork is browned and cooked through but still juicy. Serve the pork with the peanut-lime sauce on the side for dipping.
Makes 4 servings

per serving	
calories	227
total fat	6.9g
saturated fat	1.9g
cholesterol	67mg
dietary fiber	1g
carbohydrate	15g
protein	26g
sodium	375mg

good source of:
niacin, riboflavin, selenium, thiamin

ON THE *Menu*

The calories from fat for these broiled pork cutlets is under 30%, but you can improve the nutritional profile of the meal if you serve the cutlets with steamed broccoli and brown rice. For dessert, have mango sorbet and gingersnaps. All components of the meal considered, you will probably be consuming in the neighborhood of 16% calories from fat, and only 4% saturated fat.

Cincinnati Chili Casserole

Cincinnati chili was created in 1922 by a Greek restaurateur who embellished a standard American all-meat chili by adding sweet spices, such as cinnamon and allspice. He offered his customers the chili served a variety of ways, including the now well-known "five-way" chili—served on a mound of spaghetti and topped with such things as beans, chopped onions, and shredded cheese. In this baked version of Cincinnati chili, most of the components of five-way chili are combined and cooked together in a casserole.

10 ounces spaghetti
2 teaspoons olive oil
1 cup chopped onions
1 cup chopped green bell pepper
2 teaspoons minced garlic
½ pound extra-lean ground beef
½ pound ground turkey breast
2 tablespoons chili powder
1 teaspoon cinnamon
2 cups no-salt-added tomato sauce
1 tablespoon Worcestershire sauce
¾ teaspoon salt
¼ cup shredded reduced-fat Cheddar cheese

1 Preheat the oven to 400°F. Spray a 9 x 13-inch baking dish with nonstick cooking spray. In a large pot of boiling water, cook the spaghetti according to package directions. Drain.

2 Meanwhile, in a large nonstick skillet, heat the oil over medium heat. Add the onions, bell pepper, and garlic, and cook, stirring occasionally, until the onion is tender, about 10 minutes.

3 Stir in the beef, turkey, chili powder, and cinnamon, and cook, stirring, for 1 minute to coat the meat. Transfer the meat mixture to a large bowl and add the tomato sauce, Worcestershire sauce, and salt. Add the drained spaghetti, tossing to combine.

4 Transfer the mixture to the baking dish. Cover with foil and bake for 20 minutes, or until the chili is piping hot. Remove the foil, sprinkle with the Cheddar, and bake 5 minutes, or until the cheese is melted. *Makes 6 servings*

per serving	
calories	379
total fat	10g
saturated fat	3.2g
cholesterol	46mg
dietary fiber	4g
carbohydrate	48g
protein	24g
sodium	438mg

good source of: niacin, potassium, selenium, vitamin B$_{12}$, vitamin B$_6$, vitamin C, zinc

KITCHEN tip

Most supermarkets carry both "ground turkey" and "ground turkey breast." When it doesn't specify breast, it is a combination of light and dark meat and usually includes some turkey skin. Ground turkey breast is light meat and is much lower in fat. For example, 3 ounces of ground turkey breast has 0.6 grams of fat, versus 7 grams for ground turkey. If your market doesn't carry ground breast, you can grind turkey breast yourself in a food processor. Just start with chunks of turkey breast (cutlet works well) and pulse the processor on and off until the meat is fine-textured but not mushy.

Flank Steak Teriyaki

In Japanese, *teri* means shiny, and *yaki* means broil. So a teriyaki dish is one that when broiled develops a shiny glaze. To produce the glaze, traditional teriyaki sauces always contain a sweet component. For this broiled flank steak, the sweetness is provided by apple juice concentrate and a little bit of brown sugar.

3 tablespoons reduced-sodium soy sauce
2 tablespoons frozen apple juice concentrate
1 tablespoon cider vinegar
2 teaspoons light brown sugar
1 teaspoon dark sesame oil
½ teaspoon ground ginger
¼ teaspoon salt
¾ pound well-trimmed flank steak

1 In a shallow pan, stir together the soy sauce, apple juice concentrate, vinegar, brown sugar, sesame oil, ginger, and salt.

2 Add the beef, turning to coat. Refrigerate and marinate for at least 1 hour or up to overnight.

3 Preheat the broiler. Lift the beef from the marinade and place on a broiler pan. Spoon half of the marinade over the beef and broil 4 to 6 inches from the heat for 3 minutes. Spoon the remaining marinade over the beef and broil 4 to 5 minutes longer for medium-rare, or 5 to 7 minutes longer for medium. Let stand for 5 minutes before slicing on the diagonal and across the grain. ***Makes 4 servings***

Tuna Teriyaki Substitute 1 pound of tuna steak for the beef, but marinate (in the refrigerator) for 3 hours, turning the tuna over once. Broil and baste as directed, but cook for a total of 6 to 8 minutes, or until the tuna is medium-rare (cooked through but still slightly pink in the center).

per serving	
calories	176
total fat	7.8g
saturated fat	3g
cholesterol	44mg
dietary fiber	0g
carbohydrate	8g
protein	18g
sodium	603mg

good source of: vitamin B$_{12}$, zinc

ON THE *Menu*

Even though flank steak is one of the leanest cuts of beef available, it still carries with it a sizable amount of fat, so you should choose low-fat side dishes. Serve the steak with a simple whole grain (brown rice, barley, or quinoa) and Dilled Green Bean & Mushroom Salad (*page 119*). For dessert, offer Peaches & Cream (*page 136*), which sounds sinful but isn't.

Spotlite recipe

Sweet Potato & Baked Ham Salad with Ginger Dressing

Ginger juice is a wonderful, spicy ingredient with an inimitable flavor. Ordinarily, to get the juice from a ginger root you would have to grate the root and then squeeze it between your fingers to get out the juice. It's a bit labor-intensive (not to mention a bit rough on the joints), and it takes a good deal of fresh ginger to get a couple of tablespoons of juice. Luckily, there is now already-pressed juice available in bottles in the supermarket. Try it in this dressing for ham salad, but then branch out. Perk up a storebought barbecue sauce with a dash of the juice or simply stir a tablespoon into ketchup for a spicy burger topping. Or use it in a marinade made with a healthy dose of ginger juice, a little olive oil, minced garlic, and chopped cilantro.

1 pound sweet potatoes
1 can (20 ounces) juice-packed pineapple chunks, drained, ⅓ cup of juice reserved
3 tablespoons honey-mustard
2 tablespoons bottled ginger juice
2 tablespoons lime juice
2 teaspoons olive oil
½ teaspoon salt
½ teaspoon pepper
6 ounces baked ham, cut into ½-inch chunks
6 cups mixed salads greens

1 Preheat the oven to 400°F. Place the sweet potatoes on a baking sheet and bake until tender, about 45 minutes. When cool enough to handle, peel and cut into 1-inch chunks.

2 Meanwhile, in a large bowl, stir together the reserved pineapple juice, the honey-mustard, ginger juice, lime juice, oil, salt, and pepper.

3 Add the pineapple chunks, sweet potatoes, and ham, and toss to combine. Place the mixed greens on a large platter and top with the sweet potato-ham salad. *Makes 4 servings*

PER SERVING 238 calories, 5.7g total fat (0.7g saturated), 24mg cholesterol, 5g dietary fiber, 39g carbohydrate, 11g protein, 871mg sodium
Good source of: beta carotene, folate, vitamin C

F.Y.I.

Often mistaken for a wine vinegar, balsamic vinegar is actually made from highly concentrated grape juice (usually from the white Trebbiano grape) that never becomes wine, but is reduced by cooking and then aged in a succession of barrels, each from a different wood. Authentic balsamic vinegar from Italy comes in both a commercially made (*industriale*) and traditionally made (*tradizionale*) form. The commercially made vinegar is manufactured in bulk and may or may not be aged. This is the type found most commonly in supermarkets. Traditional balsamic carries a much heftier price tag, because it is always aged. The traditional should be used sparingly as it is often thick and syrupy; it is also quite expensive. Because this vinegar is so mild, you can make dressings and marinades with less oil.

Poached Orange-Basil Chicken

Though basil is a savory herb, it works well in combination with slightly sweet ingredients, like orange juice. In this low-fat chicken dish, chicken breasts are cooked in a tangy combination of orange juice, balsamic vinegar, and garlic. For a quick sauce, the poaching liquid is thickened a bit and chopped basil is stirred in.

⅔ cup orange juice
½ cup chicken broth
2 tablespoons balsamic vinegar
2 teaspoons minced garlic
½ teaspoon salt
4 skinless, boneless chicken breast halves (5 ounces each)
1½ teaspoons cornstarch blended with 1 tablespoon water
3 tablespoons chopped basil

1 In a large skillet, combine the orange juice, broth, vinegar, garlic, and salt. Bring to a boil over medium heat. Add the chicken and reduce to a simmer. Cover and cook until the chicken is cooked through, about 8 minutes.

2 Lift the chicken from the poaching liquid and transfer to serving plates. Bring the poaching liquid to a boil and stir in the cornstarch mixture. Cook, stirring, until the sauce is slightly thickened, about 1 minute. Stir in the basil. Serve the chicken with the sauce spooned on top. ***Makes 4 servings***

Pineapple-Mint Chicken In the poaching liquid (step 1), substitute pineapple juice for the orange juice, and add ⅛ teaspoon cayenne pepper. In step 2, use mint instead of basil.

Tomato-Broiled Chicken with Feta

The combination of tomato sauce and orange marmalade makes an almost instant barbecue sauce for this cheese-topped broiled chicken.

½ cup tomato sauce
½ teaspoon oregano
½ teaspoon salt
¼ teaspoon pepper
4 small skinless, boneless chicken breast halves
   (4 ounces each)
2 tablespoons orange marmalade
¼ cup crumbled feta cheese (1 ounce)

1 Preheat the broiler. In a small bowl, stir together ¼ cup of the tomato sauce, the oregano, salt, and pepper.

2 Place the chicken on a broiler pan. Brush half of the tomato mixture over the chicken breasts. Broil 4 to 6 inches from the heat for 3 minutes. Turn the chicken over, brush with the remaining tomato mixture, and broil 3 to 4 minutes or until the chicken is cooked through.

3 Meanwhile, in a small bowl, stir together the remaining ¼ cup tomato sauce and the orange marmalade.

4 Spoon the tomato-orange marmalade mixture over the chicken and sprinkle the feta on top. Broil until the feta has melted, about 1 minute.
Makes 4 servings

Crockpot cooking

By cooking the same components you'd find in chicken-noodle soup in a slow cooker, you end up with a homey, comforting stew. The results somewhat resemble a style of creamy French stew called a blanquette, which comes from the French word for white (*blanc*). In this blanquette, the chicken, mushrooms, cauliflower, and pasta all conform to the traditional color scheme, but the carrots bring a touch of color and a good helping of healthful beta carotene.

Chicken Noodle Stew with Mushrooms

2½ cups water
2 tablespoons flour
1¼ pounds skinless, boneless chicken thighs
1 cup small pasta shells or bow-tie pasta (4 ounces)
½ pound small mushrooms
2 cups fresh or 1 package (10 ounces) frozen cauliflower florets
1 cup peeled baby carrots
1 teaspoon salt
½ teaspoon rosemary

1 In a 4- or 6-quart electric slow cooker, stir the water into the flour until smooth.

2 Add the chicken, pasta, mushrooms, cauliflower, carrots, salt, and rosemary. Cover and cook on low until the chicken is tender, 6 to 8 hours. *Makes 4 servings*

PER SERVING 314 calories, 6.6g total fat (1.6g saturated), 118mg cholesterol, 4g dietary fiber, 29g carbohydrate, 34g protein, 732mg sodium
Good source of: folate, niacin, riboflavin, selenium, thiamin, vitamin B$_6$, vitamin C, zinc

Chicken with Tomatoes & Golden Raisins

This simple dish of chicken braised in a chunky fresh tomato sauce takes only about 25 minutes to cook. If you start a pot of rice at the same time, it will be ready when the chicken is done.

2 teaspoons olive oil
½ cup chopped onion
¾ cup chicken broth
3 tablespoons lemon juice
¾ teaspoon oregano
½ teaspoon salt
2 cups cherry or grape tomatoes
4 skinless, boneless chicken breast halves (5 ounces each)
¼ cup golden raisins

1 In a large nonstick skillet, heat the oil over medium heat. Add the onion and cook until tender, about 5 minutes.

2 Add the broth, lemon juice, oregano, and salt, and bring to a boil. Add the tomatoes and return to a boil.

3 Add the chicken and raisins to the pan. Reduce to a simmer and cook, uncovered, until the chicken is cooked through and the sauce is slightly thickened, about 10 minutes. ***Makes 4 servings***

Mustard-Broiled Turkey Cutlets

This simple mayonnaise-mustard topping would also work well on fish fillets or chicken cutlets.

per serving	
calories	202
total fat	5.4g
saturated fat	0.6g
cholesterol	74mg
dietary fiber	1g
carbohydrate	11g
protein	27g
sodium	838mg

good source of: niacin, selenium, vitamin B$_6$

3 tablespoons light mayonnaise
1 tablespoon Dijon mustard
1 tablespoon lemon juice
½ teaspoon salt
¼ teaspoon pepper
4 turkey cutlets (4 ounces each), halved crosswise
⅓ cup Italian-style seasoned dried breadcrumbs

1 Preheat the broiler. In a small bowl, combine the mayonnaise, mustard, lemon juice, salt, and pepper.

2 Place the turkey on a broiler pan and spread with the mayonnaise mixture. Broil the cutlets 4 to 6 inches from heat for 4 minutes, or until the cutlets are cooked through.

3 Sprinkle with the breadcrumbs and broil for 30 seconds to lightly brown the topping. ***Makes 4 servings***

Mustard-Broiled Sole Substitute 4 skinless fillets of sole (6 ounces each) for the turkey cutlets. The cooking time should be about the same, but check for doneness after 3 minutes.

ON THE *Menu*

Serve these cutlets with baked sweet potatoes, Garlicky Spinach Puree (*page 102*), and a chopped salad of tomatoes and watercress with a fat-free vinaigrette. For dessert, try Easy Rice Pudding (*page 133*).

Cajun-Style Chicken

per serving	
calories	218
total fat	4.2g
saturated fat	1.2g
cholesterol	96mg
dietary fiber	1g
carbohydrate	7g
protein	36g
sodium	414mg

good source of: niacin, selenium, vitamin B_6

Garlic powder and onion powder are common ingredients in Cajun-style cooking, where they are traditional components of the spice rub used for "blackened" food. In this recipe, they are used to season a spicy chili-sauce mixture that is spread on the chicken before broiling.

⅓ cup chili sauce
2 teaspoons Worcestershire sauce
1 teaspoon garlic powder
1 teaspoon onion powder
½ teaspoon thyme
½ teaspoon black pepper
¼ teaspoon cayenne pepper
4 skinless, boneless chicken breast halves (5 ounces each)

1 Preheat the broiler. Spray a broiler pan with nonstick cooking spray.

2 In a small bowl, combine the chili sauce, Worcestershire sauce, garlic powder, onion powder, thyme, black pepper, and cayenne.

3 Place the chicken on the broiler pan. Brush the chicken with half of the chili sauce mixture. Broil 4 to 6 inches from the heat for 4 minutes.

4 Turn the chicken over and brush evenly with the remaining chili sauce mixture. Broil for 4 minutes longer, or until the chicken is cooked. ***Makes 4 servings***

Cajun-Style Tofu Make the chili sauce mixture in step 1. Omit the chicken. Cut a 15-ounce block of extra-firm tofu in half horizontally. Brush one side of the tofu with half the chili sauce mixture and broil 4 minutes. Turn the tofu over, brush with the remaining chili sauce and broil 4 minutes until heated through and crisp on top.

F.Y.I.

A richly savory condiment based on vinegar, molasses, garlic, anchovies, tamarind, and onion, Worcestershire sauce takes its name from Worcester, England, where it was first bottled. Worcestershire is frequently served with meat—as a table condiment—but it adds an interesting sweet-savory note to sauces and marinades (or, as in this case, a spice rub). If the bottle is kept tightly capped, this potent condiment will keep almost indefinitely at room temperature.

Hunter-Style Polenta Bake

1 package (24 ounces) prepared polenta
3 tablespoons grated Parmesan cheese
10 ounces sliced roast turkey breast, torn into bite-size
   pieces
1 cup frozen peas
3 cups bottled mushroom marinara sauce

1 Preheat the oven to 425°F. Spray a 7 x 11-inch baking dish with nonstick cooking spray. Cut the polenta into 12 slices. Arrange the polenta slices, slightly overlapping, in the baking dish.

2 Sprinkle the Parmesan over the polenta. Scatter the turkey and peas over the Parmesan. Pour the marinara sauce on top. Cover with foil and bake until the polenta is piping hot and the sauce is bubbly, about 20 minutes. ***Makes 6 servings***

PER SERVING 247 calories, 1.4g total fat (0.7g saturated), 42mg cholesterol, 4g dietary fiber, 35g carbohydrate, 21g protein, 771mg sodium
Good source of: niacin, selenium

Though polenta is not difficult to make (it's only cornmeal cooked in water), it can be quite time-consuming, requiring constant stirring of the cornmeal for a good 30 minutes or so. Luckily, you can buy precooked polenta. It comes in a large sausage-shaped package and can be found in the refrigerated case of many supermarkets. With some good quality roast turkey from the deli counter and a flavorful bottled marinara sauce (we used one with mushrooms), you can have this Italian-style casserole ready to eat in about 25 minutes.

Salsa-Barbecued Chicken

Use a fairly thick bottled salsa here so it will coat the chicken well. Some storebought salsas—especially the refrigerated type—are too watery for this barbecue sauce. If your salsa seems particularly thin, you can drain it briefly in a fine-mesh sieve and then measure out 1½ cups of the drained sauce.

1½ cups bottled mild salsa
4 teaspoons chili powder
½ teaspoon oregano
4 skinless, boneless chicken breast halves (5 ounces each)
1 cup frozen corn kernels, thawed
1 tablespoon lime juice

1 In a medium bowl, stir together the salsa, chili powder, and oregano.

2 Measure out 1 cup of the salsa mixture and place it in a shallow pan big enough to hold the chicken in a single layer. Add the chicken and turn to coat well with the salsa mixture. Cover and marinate in the refrigerator for 20 minutes.

3 Meanwhile, add the corn to the bowl with the remaining salsa mixture. Stir in the lime juice.

4 Preheat the broiler. Broil the chicken 4 to 6 inches from the heat for about 8 minutes, or until cooked through. Serve the chicken with the salsa-corn mixture spooned on top. ***Makes 4 servings***

Salsa-Marinated Flank Steak Substitute 1 pound well-trimmed flank steak for the chicken. Marinate for 30 minutes in the refrigerator. Broil for about 8 minutes for medium-rare and 1 or 2 minutes longer for medium.

Orange-Baked Chicken & Couscous

The orange-flavored dried cranberries add a subtle citrus flavor to the dish, but they could be replaced by either regular dried cranberries, dried cherries, or golden raisins.

1½ teaspoons paprika
1½ teaspoons coriander
1½ teaspoons cumin
¾ teaspoon salt
1 box (10 ounces) couscous
2 teaspoons minced garlic
2 cups boiling water
4 small skinless, boneless chicken breast halves
   (4 ounces each)
⅓ cup orange-flavored dried cranberries
3 tablespoons orange all-fruit spread

1 Preheat the oven to 400°F. In a small bowl, combine the paprika, coriander, cumin, and salt. Measure out 2 teaspoons of the spice mixture to use in the couscous.

2 In a 7 x 11-inch glass baking dish, stir together the couscous and garlic. Sprinkle evenly with the reserved 2 teaspoons spice mixture. Pour the boiling water over the couscous, cover with foil, and let stand for 5 minutes.

3 Meanwhile, rub the remaining spice mixture into the chicken.

4 With a fork, stir the cranberries into the couscous. Place the chicken on top of the couscous and brush the chicken with the orange fruit spread.

5 Cover with foil and bake for 25 minutes, or until the chicken is cooked through. *Makes 4 servings*

Spotlite recipe

Grilled Duck Breast with Cherry Salsa

Skinless duck breast is actually leaner than chicken breast (120 calories and 2 grams of fat versus 140 calories and 3 grams for 3 ounces cooked). Duck can be eaten medium-rare and tastes, surprisingly, a lot like beef. Most supermarkets carry only frozen whole ducklings. But a good butcher (and even some supermarket meat departments) sell just duck breasts.

1 cup pitted cherries, thawed frozen or drained canned
⅓ cup chopped green bell pepper
⅓ cup chopped onion
3 tablespoons chili sauce
4 skinless, boneless duck breasts (5 ounces each)
¾ teaspoon salt
½ teaspoon black pepper
½ teaspoon thyme

1 In a medium bowl, stir together the cherries, bell pepper, onion, and chili sauce.

2 Spray a grill rack or stovetop grill pan with nonstick cooking spray. Preheat. Sprinkle both sides of the duck breasts with the salt, black pepper, and thyme.

3 Grill the duck breasts 4 to 6 inches from the heat, or in the pan over medium heat, until the duck is very faintly pink at the center (it will look like beef done to medium), about 3 minutes per side. When cool enough to handle, thinly slice the duck across the grain. Serve with the cherry salsa. *Makes 4 servings*

PER SERVING 201 calories, 3.1g total fat (0.7g saturated), 162mg cholesterol, 1g dietary fiber, 10g carbohydrate, 32g protein, 728mg sodium
Good source of: niacin

Chicken, Potato & Artichoke Salad

Chicken, potatoes, and artichokes are natural flavor partners in this salad tossed with a creamy lemon-tarragon dressing. The artichokes in question come in a can and are preserved in a light brine instead of the more usual high-fat vinaigrette—just check the ingredient list to be sure you're getting the right type.

> 1 pound small red potatoes
> 2 teaspoons minced garlic
> 1½ teaspoons tarragon
> ½ teaspoon salt
> 1½ cups water
> 1 pound chicken tenders
> 2 tablespoons light mayonnaise
> 1 tablespoon lemon juice
> 1 can (13¾ ounces) artichoke hearts, drained
> ½ cup jarred roasted red peppers

1 In a large pot of boiling water, cook the potatoes until tender, about 20 minutes. When cool enough to handle, thickly slice.

2 Meanwhile, in a large skillet, bring the garlic, tarragon, ¼ teaspoon of the salt, and the water to a boil over medium heat. Add the chicken, cover, and reduce to a simmer. Simmer the chicken until cooked through, about 5 minutes. Transfer the chicken to a plate, reserving the poaching liquid.

3 Transfer 1 cup of the poaching liquid to a large bowl and let cool to room temperature. Whisk in the remaining ¼ teaspoon salt, the mayonnaise, and lemon juice. Add the cooked chicken and potatoes, tossing to combine.

4 Add the artichokes and roasted peppers to the bowl with the chicken and toss to combine. Serve at room temperature or chilled. ***Makes 4 servings***

F.Y.I.

Artichokes are a good source of vitamin C, iron, potassium, magnesium, and folate. But they are an especially good source of fiber: A 2-ounce serving (the bottom of one large artichoke) has 3 grams.

Broiled Turkey with Spiced Cranberry-Pineapple Relish

If you don't have pumpkin pie spice on hand, simply combine ¼ teaspoon ground cinnamon with ⅛ teaspoon each ground allspice, nutmeg, and cloves.

⅔ cup canned whole-berry cranberry sauce
⅓ cup canned crushed pineapple
¾ teaspoon salt
½ teaspoon pumpkin pie spice
¼ teaspoon crushed red pepper flakes
I teaspoon paprika
4 turkey cutlets (4 ounces each), halved crosswise
2 teaspoons olive oil

I In a medium bowl, combine the cranberry sauce, pineapple, ¼ teaspoon of the salt, the pumpkin pie spice, and red pepper flakes. Refrigerate.

2 Preheat the broiler. Sprinkle the remaining ½ teaspoon salt and the paprika over the turkey cutlets. Brush the cutlets with the oil. Broil the cutlets 4 to 6 inches from the heat until lightly browned and cooked through, about 2 minutes per side.

3 Serve the hot cutlets with the chilled relish. *Makes 4 servings*

Broiled Pork with Cranberry-Cherry Relish In the relish, step 1, substitute cherry all-fruit spread for the crushed pineapple. Substitute 4 boneless pork loin chops (4 ounces each) for the turkey. In step 2, omit the paprika and use ½ teaspoon rubbed sage and ½ teaspoon thyme and rub them over the pork, then sprinkle with the salt.

Chicken Fingers with Honey-Mustard Sauce

When the bones are removed from a chicken breast, there's one small finger-shaped piece that hangs off the backside of the breast. This piece is called a *goujonette* in France, but in this country it is often removed from the chicken breast and sold separately as something called a chicken tender. Chicken tenders are the perfect shape for making low-fat homemade chicken fingers.

per serving	
calories	311
total fat	3.6g
saturated fat	0.8g
cholesterol	66mg
dietary fiber	1g
carbohydrate	36g
protein	33g
sodium	815mg

good source of: niacin, riboflavin, selenium, thiamin, vitamin B_6

1 cup plain dried breadcrumbs
½ teaspoon salt
¼ cup flour
¼ cup egg substitute or 2 egg whites
1 tablespoon water
1 pound chicken tenders
2 tablespoons honey
2 tablespoons Dijon mustard
1 tablespoon lemon juice

1 Preheat the oven to 450°F. Spray a large baking sheet with nonstick cooking spray.

2 On a plate, combine the breadcrumbs and salt. Place the flour on another plate. In a shallow bowl, beat the egg substitute with the water.

3 Dip the chicken first in the flour, then in the egg, and then in the breadcrumb mixture, patting it into the chicken. Place the chicken on the baking sheet and spray the chicken with nonstick cooking spray. Bake for 5 minutes, or until crisp and cooked through.

4 Meanwhile, in a medium bowl, stir together the honey, mustard, and lemon juice. Serve the chicken fingers with the honey-mustard sauce. ***Makes 4 servings***

Spicy Orange Turkey Burgers

Preformed turkey burgers are a boon to the busy cook. The spicy orange glaze brushed on these burgers gives them a special twist. If desired, top the burgers with lettuce leaves.

⅓ cup orange all-fruit spread
4 teaspoons Dijon mustard
1 tablespoon lemon juice
1½ teaspoons Louisiana-style hot sauce
¾ teaspoon salt
½ teaspoon pepper
4 packaged lean turkey burgers (4 ounces each)
4 whole-wheat hamburger buns

1 In a medium bowl, combine the orange fruit spread, mustard, lemon juice, hot sauce, ½ teaspoon of the salt, and ¼ teaspoon of the pepper. Measure out 2 tablespoons of the orange mixture and set it aside to use as a topping for the cooked burgers in step 4. Save the remainder for broiling the burgers in step 2.

2 Preheat the broiler. Sprinkle the burgers with the remaining ¼ teaspoon each salt and pepper. Spoon the remaining orange mixture over the burgers.

3 Broil the burgers 4 to 6 inches from the heat for 6 minutes, or until cooked through.

4 To serve, place the burgers on the buns and top with the reserved 2 tablespoons orange mixture. ***Makes 4 servings***

ON THE *Menu*

Although preformed turkey burgers are a convenience, they are not the lowest-fat alternative as far as ground turkey goes. So for a more balanced meal, serve the burgers with corn on the cob (skip the butter) and steamed broccoli florets. For dessert, have baked apples.

Spotlite recipe

Broiled Five-Spice Chicken

2 tablespoons plus 1 teaspoon sugar
1 tablespoon five-spice powder
¾ teaspoon salt
⅓ cup lime juice
2 tablespoons reduced-sodium soy sauce
2 teaspoons sesame oil
1 package (10 ounces) coleslaw mixture
1¼ pounds chicken tenders

1 In a large bowl, combine the sugar, five-spice powder, and salt. Measure out 5½ teaspoons of the mixture and transfer it to a medium bowl.

2 Stir the lime juice, soy sauce, and sesame oil into the spice mixture in the medium bowl. Add the coleslaw mixture and toss to combine.

3 Preheat the broiler. Add the chicken to the large bowl with the remaining spice mixture, and toss to coat. Broil the chicken 4 to 6 inches from the heat for 4 to 5 minutes, or until cooked through.

4 Serve the warm chicken on top of the slaw. *Makes 4 servings*

PER SERVING 235 calories, 6.1g total fat (1.3g saturated), 78mg cholesterol, 2g dietary fiber, 15g carbohydrate, 30g protein, 784mg sodium
Good source of: niacin, selenium, vitamin B_6, vitamin C

Tandoori-Style Turkey Cutlets

In Indian cuisine, tandoori-style dishes are those that have been baked in a high-heat clay oven called a *tandoor*. The dishes also traditionally include marinating the food first in a spiced yogurt sauce. A regular Western oven at a high temperature has to substitute for the authentic tandoor, but the marination is the same. If you like spicy food, choose a hot curry powder.

⅔ cup plain fat-free yogurt
1 tablespoon minced ginger
2 teaspoons minced garlic
2 teaspoons paprika
1½ teaspoons curry powder
½ teaspoon salt
4 turkey cutlets (4 ounces each)
¼ cup mango chutney

1 In a shallow baking pan large enough to hold the turkey cutlets in a single layer, stir together ⅓ cup of the yogurt, the ginger, garlic, paprika, curry powder, and salt. Add the turkey cutlets, turning to coat with the mixture. Cover and marinate in the refrigerator for 2 hours.

2 Preheat the oven to 450°F. Bring the turkey, in its marinade, to room temperature. Bake until the turkey is cooked through, about 10 minutes.

3 Lift the turkey from the baking pan and discard the cooked marinade. Serve the turkey with a dollop of chutney and a spoonful of the remaining ⅓ cup yogurt. ***Makes 4 servings***

F.Y.I.

Curry powder is not one spice but a blend of spices, commonly used in Indian cooking to flavor a dish with sweet heat. It also adds a characteristic yellow-orange color. While curry blends vary (consisting of as many as 20 herbs and spices), they typically include turmeric (for its vivid yellow color), fenugreek, ginger, cardamom, cloves, cumin, coriander, and cayenne pepper. Commercially available Madras curry is hotter than other store-bought types.

Maple-Mustard Chicken with Carrot Salad

Serving a cool, crunchy vegetable slaw on top of hot baked chicken breasts is an interesting contrast in temperature and textures.

> ¼ cup Dijon mustard
> ¼ cup lemon juice
> 3 tablespoons maple syrup
> ½ teaspoon tarragon
> ¼ teaspoon salt
> 4 skinless, boneless chicken breast halves (5 ounces each)
> 2 cups shredded carrots
> ¼ cup chopped onion

1 Preheat the oven to 400°F. In a medium bowl, combine the mustard, lemon juice, maple syrup, tarragon, and salt.

2 Place the chicken in a baking pan just large enough to hold it in a single layer. Spoon 6 tablespoons of the mustard mixture over the chicken. Bake until the chicken is cooked through, about 20 minutes.

3 Meanwhile, to the mustard mixture remaining in the bowl, add the carrots and onion. Toss to combine. Serve the chicken with the carrot slaw on top. *Makes 4 servings*

Off-the-Shelf

There was a time when it might have been considered unhealthful to make a dish with a can of soup, but nowadays there are lots of good low-fat, low-sodium alternatives. If you start with a low-fat soup as a base, you can "doctor it up" with herbs and a bit of cheese for a super-quick baked pasta dish.
Although this recipe assumes you have leftover chicken, you could actually just pick up some deli roast turkey and use it instead.

Mushroom-Broccoli Pasta Casserole with Chicken

8 ounces medium pasta shells
1 can (10¾ ounces) reduced-sodium, reduced-fat cream of broccoli soup
1 can (10¾ ounces) reduced-sodium, reduced-fat cream of mushroom soup
1½ cups low-fat (1%) milk
½ teaspoon rosemary, minced
2 cups shredded, cooked chicken breast (10 ounces)
⅓ cup shredded reduced-fat Cheddar cheese

1 Preheat the oven to 400°F. Spray a 7 x 11-inch baking dish with nonstick cooking spray.

2 In a large pot of boiling water, cook the pasta according to package directions. Drain.

3 Meanwhile, in a large bowl, stir together the broccoli soup, mushroom soup, milk, and rosemary. Add the pasta and chicken, and stir to combine.

4 Transfer the pasta and chicken mixture to the baking dish. Cover with foil and bake for 25 minutes, or until piping hot and bubbling. Uncover, sprinkle the Cheddar on top, and bake until the cheese has melted, about 5 minutes. *Makes 6 servings*

PER SERVING 344 calories, 6.9g total fat (2.6g saturated), 51mg cholesterol, 2g dietary fiber, 43g carbohydrate, 25g protein, 784mg sodium
Good source of: niacin, selenium

Spotlite recipe

An authentic Reuben sandwich is made with corned beef, Swiss cheese, and sauerkraut. The fat and sodium numbers for this classic New York sandwich are way off the chart. So here's a bow to the original recipe with a nutrition profile that is much more laudable. Roast turkey replaces the fatty corned beef and fresh coleslaw mix replaces the high-sodium sauerkraut. For an interesting twist, the sandwich is spread with cranberry mayonnaise, making it a good option for Thanksgiving leftovers.

Roast Turkey "Reuben"

⅓ cup whole-berry cranberry sauce
1 tablespoon light mayonnaise
8 slices rye bread, toasted
6 ounces sliced roast turkey breast
1⅓ cups packaged coleslaw mixture
4 slices (½ ounce each) reduced-fat Swiss cheese

1 Preheat the broiler. In a small bowl, stir together the cranberry sauce and mayonnaise.

2 Place 4 slices of the toast on a broiler pan and spread with the cranberry sauce-mayonnaise mixture. Top each piece of toast with the turkey. Top with the coleslaw mix. Top with the Swiss cheese.

3 Broil 4 to 6 inches from the heat until the cheese has melted, about 1 minute. Top with the remaining 4 slices toast. *Makes 4 servings*

PER SERVING 300 calories, 6.5g total fat (2.6g saturated), 47mg cholesterol, 4g dietary fiber, 40g carbohydrate, 22g protein, 449mg sodium
Good source of: niacin, selenium

Fusilli with Herbed Winter Squash Sauce

Winter squash puree, with its velvety texture and subtle, sweet flavor, makes a rich, quick, and easy topping for pasta.

12 ounces short fusilli, penne, or ziti pasta
¾ cup evaporated low-fat (2%) milk
2 tablespoons sugar
1 teaspoon salt
¼ teaspoon pepper
¼ teaspoon rubbed sage
1 package (12 ounces) frozen winter squash puree, thawed
3 tablespoons grated Parmesan cheese

1 In a large pot of boiling water, cook the fusilli according to package directions. Drain, reserving 1 cup of the pasta cooking water.

2 Meanwhile, in a large skillet, combine the evaporated milk, sugar, salt, pepper, and sage. Bring to a boil over medium heat. Add the winter squash and bring to a simmer.

3 Transfer the winter squash puree to a large bowl and stir in the reserved pasta cooking water and the Parmesan. Add the pasta and toss to coat. *Makes 4 servings*

Brown Rice & Winter Squash "Risotto" Omit the pasta. Cook 2 cups of brown rice according to package directions. In step 2, increase the evaporated milk to 1 cup and add ½ cup of water. In step 3, increase the Parmesan to ¼ cup and omit the pasta cooking water. Stir the cooked brown rice into the sauce.

Couscous with Carrots & Chick-Peas

The combination of couscous and chick-peas makes an immensely satisfying meatless main dish. All you need to round out the meal is a tossed salad and maybe a scoop of fruit sorbet for dessert.

2¼ cups water
1 tablespoon olive oil
2 teaspoons minced garlic
1½ teaspoons paprika
¾ teaspoon salt
¼ teaspoon pepper
1 box (10 ounces) couscous
1 cup shredded carrots
1 can (15½ ounces) chick-peas, rinsed and drained
¾ cup dried currants or raisins

F.Y.I.

Couscous can now be found in a range of colors and flavors, much like other pastas. You may be able to find tomato, spinach, or tri-color versions. Any one of them would be good in this recipe.

1 In a large saucepan, combine the water, oil, garlic, paprika, salt, and pepper. Bring to a boil over high heat.

2 Stir in the couscous and carrots, and remove from the heat. Cover and let stand for 5 minutes.

3 Uncover and fluff the couscous with a fork. Stir in the chick-peas and currants. *Makes 4 servings*

Chicken Couscous In step 1, reduce the water to 1¼ cups and add 1 cup of chicken broth. Cook the couscous as directed. When fluffing the couscous, add 1½ cups cut-up cooked chicken or turkey breast. Stir in the chick-peas and currants, but reduce the currants to ¼ cup.

Off-the-Shelf

This four-ingredient dish is way more than the sum of its parts. And the mere 10 minutes it takes to put together (not counting the time is takes to bring the gnocchi cooking water to a boil) only makes the interesting and flavorful results more surprising.

Potato Gnocchi with Pesto-Broccoli Sauce

1 package (25 ounces) potato gnocchi
1 can (10¾ ounces) reduced-sodium, reduced-fat
    cream of broccoli soup
½ cup low-fat (1%) milk
3 tablespoons storebought pesto

1 In a large pot of boiling water, cook the gnocchi according to package directions. Drain, reserving ½ cup of the cooking water. Transfer the gnocchi to a bowl.

2 Meanwhile, in a small saucepan, heat the soup and milk over low heat. Stir in the reserved cooking water and the pesto.

3 Pour the soup mixture over the gnocchi, and toss to combine. *Makes 6 servings*

PER SERVING 331 calories, 6.8g total fat (2.3g saturated), 14mg cholesterol, 3g dietary fiber, 57g carbohydrate, 11g protein, 891mg sodium

Spotlite recipe

The beauty of layered salads is that you can assem-
ble them well ahead of
time. And because the
ingredients are not tossed
with the dressing until the
last minute, they remain
crisp and unwilted. The
classic American layered
salad (a favorite at potluck
dinners and backyard bar-
becues) is called Peas &
Cheese. We've taken that
as our inspiration, but
given it a European twist
by using Mediterranean-
style salad mix (which
usually includes some
interesting salad greens
such as radicchio), chick-
peas instead of the traditional green peas, and
Greek feta instead of Cheddar cheese.

Mediterranean Peas & Cheese Salad

1 cup plain fat-free yogurt
1/3 cup fat-free sour cream
1 tablespoon lemon juice
1 teaspoon dillweed
1 teaspoon dried lemon peel
2 cans (15 1/2 ounces each) chick-peas, rinsed and
   drained
1 pint grape tomatoes
4 1/2 cups Mediterranean salad mix
1/2 cup crumbled reduced-fat feta cheese (2 ounces)

1 In a small bowl, combine the yogurt, sour cream, lemon juice, dillweed, and lemon peel.

2 In an 8- to 10-cup glass bowl, arrange the chick-peas, tomatoes, and salad mix in layers, ending with the salad mix. Pour the yogurt mixture over the salad mix and sprinkle with the feta cheese. Cover well and refrigerate for at least 1 hour or up to overnight.

3 At serving time, toss the salad. **Makes 4 servings**

PER SERVING 282 calories, 5.4g total fat (1.6g saturated), 6mg cholesterol, 11g dietary fiber, 44g carbohydrate, 17g protein, 627mg sodium
Good source of: fiber, folate, vitamin C

Chili Rice & Beans

The combination of rice and beans provides a good amount of protein in this meatless main dish. For a completely vegetarian version, substitute vegetable broth for the chicken broth.

per serving	
calories	344
total fat	6.1g
saturated fat	1.1g
cholesterol	2mg
dietary fiber	8g
carbohydrate	62g
protein	11g
sodium	545mg

good source of: fiber, folate, thiamin, vitamin C

1 tablespoon olive oil
¾ cup chopped onion
1 cup chopped green bell pepper
4 cloves garlic, minced
1 cup rice
1 tablespoon chili powder
1½ cups chicken broth
¾ cup water
1 can (19 ounces) red kidney beans, rinsed and drained

1 In a medium saucepan, heat the oil over medium heat. Add the onion, bell pepper, and garlic, and cook, stirring occasionally, until the onion is tender, about 7 minutes.

2 Add the rice, chili powder, broth, and water, and bring to a boil. Reduce to a simmer, cover, and cook for 17 minutes or until the rice is tender.

3 Stir in the beans and cook until heated through, about 2 minutes. ***Makes 4 servings***

Golden Rice & Black Beans In step 2, omit the chicken broth and reduce the water to ¼ cup. Add 2 cups carrot juice and cook the rice as directed. In step 3, use black beans instead of kidney beans and add ¾ teaspoon salt and ¼ teaspoon black pepper.

F.Y.I.

Anchovy paste is a combination of mashed anchovies, vinegar, spices, and water and is most often sold in convenient tubes. It's a quick, easy way to infuse sauces and marinades with robust flavor and only minimal fat—if used sparingly. Store the tube in the refrigerator after opening it.

Penne with Spicy Broccoli Sauce

Chopped broccoli makes a surprisingly good (and healthful) pasta sauce. Delicious hot, this pasta dish can also be served at room temperature.

    10 ounces whole-wheat penne
    1 tablespoon olive oil
    1 cup chopped onion
    1 tablespoon minced garlic
    1 tablespoon anchovy paste
    ½ teaspoon crushed red pepper flakes
    2 packages (10 ounces each) frozen chopped broccoli,
        thawed
    ½ teaspoon salt
    ⅓ cup grated Parmesan cheese

1 In a large pot of boiling water, cook the pasta according to package directions. Drain, reserving 1 cup of the pasta cooking water.

2 Meanwhile, in a large nonstick skillet, heat the oil over medium heat. Add the onion and garlic, and cook, stirring frequently, until the onion is tender, about 7 minutes.

3 Add the anchovy paste and red pepper flakes, and cook until the anchovy paste has melted, about 1 minute.

4 Add the broccoli and salt, and cook until the broccoli is tender, about 3 minutes. Transfer to a large serving bowl. Add the reserved pasta cooking water, the pasta, and the Parmesan, and toss to combine. *Makes 4 servings*

Radiatore with Spicy Cauliflower Sauce Use radiatore pasta instead of penne. Substitute 2 packages of frozen cauliflower florets for the broccoli. Add ¼ cup of dried currants when adding the cauliflower in step 4.

Crockpot cooking

In an ordinary stew, you **would** have to presoak the dried mushrooms before using them. But because this tomato-y cannellini and barley stew is slow-cooked, all you have to do is rinse the mushrooms under running water to wash off any grit. The combination of mushrooms, beans, and barley provide plenty of dietary fiber (over 50% of the recommended intake), with nearly 25% of that being heart-healthy soluble fiber.

White Bean & Barley Stew

½ cup dried mushroom pieces or slices
2 cans (15½ ounces each) cannellini beans, rinsed and drained
¾ cup pearl barley
1 can (14½ ounces) stewed tomatoes
¾ cup carrot juice
1¾ cups water
1 tablespoon minced garlic
½ teaspoon salt
½ teaspoon pepper
½ teaspoon marjoram or oregano

1 In a strainer, rinse the mushrooms under running water.

2 In a 4- or 6-quart electric slow cooker, combine the rinsed mushrooms, beans, barley, stewed tomatoes, carrot juice, water, garlic, salt, pepper, and marjoram.

3 Cook on low until the barley is tender, 6 to 8 hours. *Makes 4 servings*

PER SERVING **389 calories, 1.1g total fat (0.3g saturated), 0mg cholesterol, 17g dietary fiber, 79g carbohydrate, 18g protein, 903mg sodium**
Good source of: **beta carotene, fiber, folate, magnesium, potassium, selenium, vitamin B$_6$, zinc**

Asparagus & Cheese Strata

Stratas are basically savory, layered French toast. Slices of bread (toasted for extra flavor) are layered with other ingredients—here it's asparagus and cheese—and then soaked with a custard. When the strata bakes, the cheese melts and the bread layer puffs up and browns. Best of all, the strata is designed to be assembled way ahead of baking. You could put it together in the morning and then refrigerate it until an hour or so before dinner.

per serving	
calories	274
total fat	6.3g
saturated fat	3g
cholesterol	13mg
dietary fiber	5g
carbohydrate	34g
protein	22g
sodium	822mg

good source of:
riboflavin, selenium, vitamin B$_{12}$

8 slices (1 ounce each) 7-grain or whole-wheat bread, toasted
1 can (10½ ounces) cut asparagus spears, drained
½ cup shredded reduced-fat Cheddar cheese
2 tablespoons grated Parmesan cheese
2 cups fat-free milk
1 cup (8 ounces) egg substitute or 8 large egg whites
½ teaspoon salt
½ teaspoon oregano

1 Spray a 9-inch square baking dish with nonstick cooking spray. Arrange 4 of the bread slices in a single layer in the dish. Scatter the asparagus over the bread. Sprinkle the Cheddar and Parmesan over the asparagus.

2 In a large bowl, stir together the milk, egg substitute, salt, and oregano. Place the remaining 4 slices of bread on top. Pour the egg mixture over the bread. Cover and refrigerate for at least 30 minutes, and up to overnight.

3 Preheat the oven to 350°F. Bake the strata, uncovered, for 45 minutes, or until the top is golden brown and a knife inserted in the center comes out clean. *Makes 4 servings*

Mexican Corn & Pepper Strata Substitute a can of Mexican corn for the asparagus. Substitute jack cheese for the Cheddar. Add 1 tablespoon chili powder to the milk mixture in step 2.

Tortellini with Zesty Red Pepper Sauce

You can prepare the sauce ahead of time (using ¾ cup of water instead of the pasta cooking water) and refrigerate it. Then gently reheat the sauce while the pasta cooks.

1 package (15 ounces) frozen cheese tortellini
1 cup jarred roasted red peppers, drained
1 can (6 ounces) tomato paste
2 teaspoons minced garlic
½ teaspoon salt
½ teaspoon ground ginger
¼ teaspoon cayenne pepper
½ cup orange juice
1 package (10 ounces) frozen peas, thawed

1 In a large pot of boiling water, cook the tortellini according to package directions. Drain, reserving ¾ cup of the pasta cooking water.

2 Meanwhile, in a food processor, combine the roasted peppers, tomato paste, garlic, salt, ginger, and cayenne, and puree until smooth.

3 Transfer the sauce to a large skillet and add the reserved pasta cooking water, the orange juice, and the peas. Bring to a boil over medium heat.

4 Pour the sauce into a serving bowl. Add the hot tortellini and toss to combine. ***Makes 4 servings***

Tortellini with Yellow Pepper-Basil Sauce In step 2, substitute 2 cups jarred roasted yellow peppers for the red. Omit the tomato paste, garlic, and ginger and use 2 tablespoons storebought pesto instead.

KITCHEN *tip*

You can also make the sauce as described in step 2 only (that is, without thinning it with water or orange juice) and serve it as a dipping sauce for vegetables or chips.

Off-the-Shelf

Easy Salsa Pasta

10 ounces ziti or penne pasta
1 package (10 ounces) frozen corn kernels
1 can (15½ ounces) black beans, rinsed and drained
1 cup bottled mild to medium salsa
⅓ cup shredded Mexican cheese blend
2 teaspoons olive oil

1   In a large pot of boiling water, cook the pasta according to package directions. Add the corn for the last 30 seconds of cooking to thaw. Drain.

2   Transfer the drained pasta and corn to a large bowl. Add the black beans, salsa, cheese, and oil, and toss to combine. ***Makes 4 servings***

PER SERVING 443 calories, 7.2g total fat (2.4g saturated), 8mg cholesterol, 10g dietary fiber, 79g carbohydrate, 18g protein, 510mg sodium
Good source of: **fiber, folate, niacin, selenium, thiamin**

Bottled salsa makes a super-quick pasta sauce, but be sure to use one that is fairly thick or the sauce will be too watery. Generally speaking, the refrigerated salsas are the more watery types. As to the cheese for this pasta dish, most supermarkets carry what is labeled Mexican cheese blend, which is usually a mixture of Monterey jack, Cheddar, and often a mild white cheese similar to a Mexican *queso bianco*.

Spinach & Mushroom Pizza

An Italian prebaked pizza crust—the type commonly available in supermarkets—gets topped with spinach, mushrooms, and a mixture of fresh cheeses and Parmesan.

1 large (12 inches) prebaked thin Italian pizza crust
⅔ cup tomato sauce
⅔ cup fat-free cottage cheese
½ cup part-skim ricotta cheese
2 tablespoons grated Parmesan cheese
½ teaspoon garlic powder
1 package (10 ounces) frozen chopped spinach, thawed
   and drained
1½ cups sliced mushrooms (6 ounces)

1 Preheat the oven to 450°F. Place the pizza crust on a large baking sheet. Spread the tomato sauce on the crust.

2 In a medium bowl, combine the cottage cheese, ricotta, Parmesan, and garlic powder. Spread the cheese mixture on the pizza crust. Top with the spinach and mushrooms, and bake for 10 minutes, or until heated through.
Makes 4 servings

Pepper & Onion Pizza Omit the spinach and mushrooms. Top the cheese mixture in step 2 with 1½ cups jarred roasted red or yellow peppers (cut into strips) and 1½ cups chopped onions.

Pasta with Spinach Pesto

Use this spinach pesto in other dishes, too. For example, make a double batch of the sauce (using 1 cup of water instead of the pasta cooking water called for below), and spoon it over grilled chicken or fish or toss it with hot cooked potatoes. The pesto will keep for several days in the refrigerator.

12 ounces penne pasta
1 package (10 ounces) frozen spinach, thawed and drained
¼ cup chopped basil
¼ cup walnut pieces
2 teaspoons minced garlic
2 tablespoons light mayonnaise
3 tablespoons grated Parmesan cheese
½ teaspoon salt

1 In a large pot of boiling water, cook the pasta according to package directions. Drain, reserving ½ cup of the pasta cooking water.

2 In a food processor, combine the spinach, basil, walnuts, garlic, mayonnaise, Parmesan, and salt, and puree until smooth.

3 Transfer the pesto to a large bowl, add the reserved pasta cooking water and the pasta, and toss to combine. ***Makes 4 servings***

KITCHEN *tip*

Jars of pre-chopped basil are available in the supermarket. The basil is packed in water and can usually be found in the refrigerated section of the produce department.

Off-the-Shelf

Mushroom-Asparagus Lasagna

2 cans (10¾ ounces each) reduced-sodium, reduced-fat cream of mushroom soup
1 can (12 ounces) evaporated fat-free milk
¾ teaspoon tarragon
½ teaspoon pepper
12 pieces oven-ready lasagna (from an 8-ounce package)
1 package (10 ounces) frozen asparagus spears, thawed
2 cups (8 ounces) shredded fat-free mozzarella
4 teaspoons sliced almonds
2 tablespoons grated Parmesan cheese

1 Preheat the oven to 375°F. In a medium bowl, stir together the soup, evaporated milk, tarragon, and pepper. Spoon ½ cup of the soup mixture into the bottom of a 9 x 13-inch baking pan.

2 Place 3 pieces of uncooked lasagna over the sauce, without overlapping or touching the sides of the pan since they will expand as they bake. Top the pasta with one-third of the asparagus, ⅓ cup of the mozzarella, and ¾ cup of the soup mixture. Repeat this layering two more times.

3 Top with the remaining 3 pieces of lasagna, remaining soup, and 1 cup mozzarella. Sprinkle the almonds and Parmesan on top.

4 Cover with foil. Bake for 30 minutes. Remove the foil and bake for 10 to 15 minutes, or until hot and bubbling. Let stand for 5 minutes before cutting. ***Makes 6 servings***

PER SERVING **333 calories, 6.9g total fat (2g saturated), 17mg cholesterol, 3g dietary fiber, 44g carbohydrate, 25g protein, 406mg sodium**
Good source of: **calcium, folate, riboflavin, selenium**

Crockpot cooking

Chick-Pea & Butternut Stew

2 cups dried chick-peas, rinsed and picked over
3 cups water
1 cup chopped onion
1 cup chopped green bell pepper
2 cups frozen butternut squash chunks
1 can (15½ ounces) crushed tomatoes
1 tablespoon minced garlic
1½ teaspoons paprika
1¼ teaspoons coriander
1 teaspoon salt
¼ teaspoon cayenne pepper

Because the chick-peas are being cooked from scratch, you have to start them out on their own, cooking them at high heat. So if you're making this for dinner, start the chick-peas cooking in the morning. After the chick-peas have cooked for about 1 hour, add the other ingredients and let them cook on low heat until dinner time. As the butternut squash cooks, it breaks down and forms the basis for a smooth tomato-vegetable sauce.

1 In a large bowl, combine the chick-peas and water to cover by several inches. Let stand at room temperature overnight. Drain.

2 In a 4- or 6-quart electric slow cooker, combine the drained chick-peas and 1½ cups of the water, and cook on high heat for 1 hour.

3 Add the onion, bell pepper, squash, tomatoes, garlic, paprika, coriander, salt, and cayenne.

4 Add the remaining 1½ cups water. Stir to combine. Cook on low heat until the chick-peas are tender, about 8 hours. *Makes 6 servings*

PER SERVING 293 calories, 4.1g total fat (0.4g saturated), 0mg cholesterol, 15g dietary fiber, 54g carbohydrate, 15g protein, 498mg sodium
Good source of: beta carotene, fiber, folate, magnesium, potassium, thiamin, vitamin B$_6$, vitamin C

per serving	
calories	198
total fat	4.7g
saturated fat	0.7g
cholesterol	0mg
dietary fiber	4g
carbohydrate	36g
protein	4g
sodium	303mg

good source of: niacin, potassium, thiamin, vitamin B_6, vitamin C

F.Y.I.

Roasting does not affect the potassium content of potatoes, which are an excellent source of this mineral. Potassium is vital for many functions, including protein synthesis from amino acids and carbohydrate metabolism. In addition, potassium is necessary for the building of muscle and for normal body growth. The vitamin C in potatoes, however, is partially destroyed by the high heat of roasting.

Herb-Roasted New Potatoes & Garlic

The potatoes used in this recipe are commonly called new potatoes, although that is just a term used in markets to describe all thin-skinned "boiling" potatoes. (Real "new" potatoes are actually those that have been freshly dug and have not been stored.) Boiling potatoes have a denser, waxier flesh than typical dry-fleshed baking potatoes (such as Idahos).

> 2 tablespoons olive oil
> 12 cloves garlic, unpeeled
> 1 bay leaf
> ¾ teaspoon rosemary
> ½ teaspoon thyme
> 2 pounds very small red or white potatoes
> ¾ teaspoon salt

1 Preheat the oven to 425°F. In a 9 x 13-inch baking pan, combine the olive oil, garlic, bay leaf, rosemary, and thyme.

2 Add the potatoes and toss to coat. Bake for 45 minutes, or until the potatoes are tender and the skin is lightly crisped.

3 Remove and discard the bay leaf. Sprinkle the salt over the potatoes and serve them with the garlic cloves. (The garlic cloves will be soft and mild-flavored, and can easily be squeezed out of their skin and eaten with the potatoes.) *Makes 6 servings*

per serving	
calories	209
total fat	1.9g
saturated fat	0.5g
cholesterol	2mg
dietary fiber	6g
carbohydrate	41g
protein	7g
sodium	369mg

good source of: fiber

Mushroom-Topped Mashed Potatoes

For a real treat, try this recipe with a combination of dried porcini mushrooms and sliced fresh button mushrooms. Use about ½ pound of button mushrooms, and ½ cup dried porcini. Reconstitute the porcini in a bowl of very hot water for about 20 minutes to soften them. Scoop the mushrooms out of the soaking water so that any dirt clinging to them will be left behind in the bowl. Add the dried and fresh mushrooms all at the same time, in step 1.

2 teaspoons olive oil
¾ pound sliced portobello mushrooms
3 teaspoons minced garlic
¾ teaspoon salt
¼ cup plus ⅔ cup water
1 cup low-fat (1%) milk
1⅓ cups instant mashed potato flakes
2 tablespoons fat-free sour cream

1   In a large nonstick skillet, heat the oil over medium heat. Add the mushrooms, 1 teaspoon of the garlic, ¼ teaspoon of the salt, and ¼ cup of the water. Cover and cook until the mushrooms are tender, about 7 minutes.

2   Meanwhile, in a medium saucepan, bring the milk, the remaining ⅔ cup water, 2 teaspoons garlic, and ½ teaspoon salt to a simmer over medium heat. Remove from the heat and stir in the mashed potato flakes until evenly moistened.

2   Stir the sour cream into the mashed potatoes. Serve the potatoes topped with the mushrooms. *Makes 6 servings*

F.Y.I.

Fragrant, flavorful dark (toasted) sesame oil contains monounsaturated and polyunsaturated fats as well as vitamin E. To prevent sesame oil from going rancid, keep it refrigerated.

Sesame-Roasted Asparagus

Although many people prize skinny stalks of asparagus (sometimes referred to as "pencil grass"), they are not a good choice when it comes to roasting. For this dish, choose spears that are at least ½ inch in diameter.

> ½ cup water
> 2 teaspoons dark sesame oil
> 1 tablespoon reduced-sodium soy sauce
> 1¼ pounds asparagus

1 Preheat the oven to 450°F. In a 9 x 13-inch baking pan, combine the water, sesame oil, and soy sauce. Add the asparagus and toss well to coat.

2 Place in the oven and roast uncovered for 20 minutes, or until the water has evaporated and the asparagus are tender and lightly browned. Serve hot or at room temperature. *Makes 4 servings*

Roasted Green Beans Substitute 1¼ pounds flat Italian green beans or regular green beans for the asparagus.

Garlicky Spinach Puree

Cream of rice is the secret ingredient in this puree, adding thickness and a creamy texture with no fat. To drain the spinach, set it out to thaw in a strainer set in the sink or over a bowl. As it starts to come to room temperature, use a fork to break up the chunks of spinach. This will make it easier for the liquid to drain off.

per serving	
calories	99
total fat	3.2g
saturated fat	1g
cholesterol	5mg
dietary fiber	4g
carbohydrate	13g
protein	7g
sodium	579mg

good source of: beta carotene, calcium, fiber, folate, magnesium, potassium, riboflavin, thiamin, vitamin B_{12}, vitamin B_6, vitamin C, vitamin E

1½ teaspoons olive oil
4 teaspoons minced garlic
2 packages (10 ounces each) frozen chopped spinach, thawed and drained
4 teaspoons cream of rice
1 cup fat-free milk
¾ teaspoon salt
2 tablespoons reduced-fat sour cream

1 In a large nonstick skillet, heat the oil over low heat. Add the garlic and cook until tender, about 2 minutes. Stir in the spinach and cook 3 minutes.

2 Sprinkle the cream of rice over the spinach and cook, stirring, for 2 minutes. Add the milk and salt and simmer, stirring occasionally, until slightly thickened, about 3 minutes.

3 Transfer the mixture to a food processor. Add the sour cream and puree until smooth. *Makes 4 servings*

Crockpot cooking

Baked beans are a natural for a slow cooker. In a traditional baked bean recipe, small white beans are cooked in a ceramic bean pot in a very low oven for hours. The cook has to keep an eye on the beans, adding liquid now and again to be sure the beans don't bake dry. The electric slow cooker solves the problem by keeping the moisture in. We've also streamlined the process by starting with canned beans, since dried beans have to be soaked overnight before you can cook them. Most of the flavors of a traditional baked bean dish are still here, though, including a splash of rum or bourbon. The only obvious omission is the piece of pork fatback that is usually included.

Crockpot Baked Beans

3 cans (15 ounces each) pinto beans, rinsed and
  drained
⅔ cup canned crushed tomatoes
½ cup chopped onion
⅓ cup packed light brown sugar
3 tablespoons dark rum or bourbon
2 tablespoons Dijon mustard
½ teaspoon thyme
½ teaspoon ground ginger
½ teaspoon salt

1 In a 4- or-6-quart electric slow cooker, combine the beans, tomatoes, onion, brown sugar, rum, mustard, thyme, ginger, and salt.

2 Cook on low until the beans have absorbed most of the liquid and are rich and flavorful, 4 to 6 hours. *Makes 8 servings*

PER SERVING 181 calories, 0.9g total fat (0.1g saturated), 0mg cholesterol, 8g dietary fiber, 34g carbohydrate, 8g protein, 518mg sodium
Good source of: fiber, folate, potassium, thiamin

Hot & Sour Collards & Corn

Seasoning cooked greens with vinegar and hot sauce is typical of Southern cooking. Of course, a Southern greens dish would also include a ham hock or some other high-fat smoked meat. We've made this a much more healthful dish by adding just a bit of liquid smoke seasoning instead. While we've used all collard greens, you could use a mixture of collards and kale or any sturdy cooking greens.

2 tablespoons water
2 teaspoons olive oil
2 packages (16 ounces each) frozen chopped collards, thawed
¾ teaspoon salt
1½ cups frozen corn kernels
2 tablespoons red wine vinegar
2 teaspoons Louisiana-style hot sauce
½ teaspoon liquid smoke seasoning

1 In a large nonstick skillet, bring the water and oil to a simmer over medium heat. Add the collards and stir to combine. Add the salt, cover, and cook, stirring occasionally, until the collards are tender, about 25 minutes.

2 Stir in the corn, vinegar, hot sauce, and liquid smoke, and cook until the corn is heated through, about 3 minutes. ***Makes 4 servings***

per serving	
calories	156
total fat	3.7g
saturated fat	0.5g
cholesterol	0mg
dietary fiber	8g
carbohydrate	29g
protein	9g
sodium	614mg

good source of: beta carotene, calcium, fiber, folate, magnesium, niacin, potassium, riboflavin, vitamin B_6, vitamin C

F.Y.I.

Liquid smoke is a seasoning liquid made from water and concentrated smoke. A small amount of liquid smoke adds a flavor that mimics that found in smoked meats, giving a traditional taste to such dishes as split pea soup, braised greens, and baked beans without adding any saturated fat. The most common liquid smoke is made from hickory, but other woods are available, such as mesquite.

Baked Mushrooms & Corn

This is a really easy side dish. It involves only about 5 minutes of preparation (if you buy presliced mushrooms) before you put the dish in the oven. The rest of preparation time is unattended cooking, while the vegetables bake in the oven.

> 1 pound sliced mushrooms
> 1 package (10 ounces) frozen corn kernels
> ½ cup chopped onion
> 1 teaspoon minced garlic
> 1 teaspoon chili powder
> ¾ teaspoon sugar
> ½ teaspoon salt
> 2 teaspoons olive oil

1 Preheat the oven to 400°F. In a 9 x 13-inch baking pan, toss together the mushrooms, corn, onion, garlic, chili powder, sugar, and salt. Drizzle with the oil and toss again.

2 Bake until the mushrooms and onions are tender, about 20 minutes. Serve warm or at room temperature. ***Makes 4 servings***

Mushroom, Corn & Onion Pizza Make the baked mushrooms and corn as directed. Leave the oven on. Brush 1 large (12 inches) prebaked thin pizza crust with ¼ cup tomato paste. Scatter 1 cup chopped onions on top. Top with the baked mushrooms and corn, and sprinkle with 2 tablespoons grated Parmesan. Bake for 10 minutes.

F.Y.I.

Cauliflower is a good source of the B vitamin folate and vitamin B_6. Because B vitamins are water-soluble, it's always best to cook cauliflower in such a way that these vitamins are not thrown away with the cooking water. In this puree, the cauliflower is cooked in milk, which is then used in the puree, so the B vitamins are preserved.

Cauliflower, Potato & Cheese Puree

Vegetable purees are vastly underrated side dishes. They are easy to make and have an extremely comforting texture. This mixture of cauliflower and mashed potatoes is rich with two cheeses and garlic.

⅔ cup fat-free milk
1 teaspoon minced garlic
½ teaspoon salt
¼ teaspoon marjoram or thyme
⅛ teaspoon cayenne pepper
1 package (10 ounces) frozen cauliflower, thawed
¼ cup instant mashed potato flakes
¼ cup shredded reduced-fat Cheddar cheese
1 tablespoon grated Parmesan cheese

1 In a medium saucepan, combine the milk, garlic, salt, marjoram, and cayenne. Bring to a simmer over low heat. Add the cauliflower, cover, and cook until the cauliflower is tender, about 5 minutes.

2 Transfer the cauliflower mixture to a food processor. Add the instant mashed potatoes, Cheddar, and Parmesan, and puree. Serve hot. ***Makes 4 servings***

Cauliflower, Potato & Cheese Soup In step 1, increase the marjoram and cayenne to ½ teaspoon each, and increase the salt to 1 teaspoon. In step 2, when pureeing the vegetables, add 1⅔ cups of fat-free milk to thin the puree to soup consistency. If necessary, reheat the soup gently.

Oven-Braised Baby Zucchini

Baby zucchini are a wonderful convenience, because you don't have to peel them or cut them up. Just pop them in a baking dish, season or sauce them, and you have a delicious side dish. However, baby zucchini are seasonal, so when they are not available, substitute the smallest zucchini you can find and halve them lengthwise.

1 can (14½ ounces) stewed tomatoes
¼ cup orange juice
¼ teaspoon salt
1¼ pounds baby zucchini (about 12)
¼ cup plain dried breadcrumbs
2 tablespoons grated Parmesan cheese

1 Preheat the oven to 400°F. In a 7 x 11-inch baking dish, combine the tomatoes, orange juice, and salt.

2 Top with the zucchini, cover with foil, and bake for 45 minutes, or until the zucchini are tender.

3 Uncover. Scatter the breadcrumbs and Parmesan evenly over the top and bake for 5 minutes, or until the crumbs are golden brown. *Makes 4 servings*

Tomato-Braised Zucchini & Beans For a hearty vegetarian main dish, use 1 can (15 ounces) of rinsed and drained chick-peas or white beans and stir them in with the tomatoes in step 1.

Mint-Glazed Brussels Sprouts

Mint-flavored jelly makes a surprisingly delicious glaze for Brussels sprouts. The water chestnuts, too, take on the sweet-tart-herbal flavor. If you can't find diced water chestnuts, simply use sliced.

2 packages (10 ounces each) frozen Brussels sprouts
2 teaspoons olive oil
1 can (11 ounces) diced water chestnuts, drained
⅓ cup mint-flavored apple jelly
2 tablespoons cider vinegar
1 teaspoon coriander
¾ teaspoon salt

1 In a large pot of boiling water, cook the Brussels sprouts until crisp-tender, about 7 minutes. Drain.

2 In a large nonstick skillet, heat the oil over medium heat. Add the Brussels sprouts, water chestnuts, jelly, vinegar, coriander, and salt. Increase the heat to high and cook until the Brussels sprouts are nicely glazed and tender, about 10 minutes. ***Makes 4 servings***

Mint-Glazed Cherry Tomatoes Use 2 pints of cherry or grape tomatoes instead of the Brussels sprouts and omit step 1. Use lemon juice instead of vinegar in step 2.

F.Y.I.

Brussels sprouts belong to the family of cruciferous vegetables, which contain indoles, phytochemicals that are thought to have cancer-fighting potential. They are also a rich source of fiber and provide a good amount of vitamin C (1 cup has 108% of the RDA for men).

Off-the-Shelf

Storebought pesto is a
great ingredient to keep
around for an easy boost
to the flavor of pasta
sauces, soups, stews,
mashed potatoes, salad
dressings, or a vegetable
side dish such as these Italian beans. Although storebought versions of this
delicious basil, cheese, and
garlic sauce are no light-
weights in the fat department, just 1 tablespoon will
make a significant flavor
contribution to a dish.

Garlic-Basil Italian Beans

¼ cup water

2 teaspoons minced garlic

2 packages (10 ounces each) frozen Italian green
    beans, thawed

1 can (14½ ounces) diced tomatoes

½ teaspoon salt

½ teaspoon dried lemon peel or 1 teaspoon grated fresh
    lemon zest

1 tablespoon storebought pesto

1 In a large skillet, bring the water and minced garlic to a boil over
medium heat. Cook until the garlic is tender and the water has evaporated, about 3 minutes.

2 Add the green beans, tomatoes, salt, and lemon peel, and cook until the
beans are tender and the sauce has reduced slightly, about 7 minutes. Stir
in the pesto and serve hot. *Makes 4 servings*

PER SERVING **88 calories, 2.3g total fat (0.5g saturated), 1mg cholesterol,
5g dietary fiber, 16g carbohydrate, 4g protein, 474mg sodium**
Good source of: **calcium, fiber, magnesium, potassium, riboflavin, thiamin,
vitamin B$_6$, vitamin C, vitamin E**

Smashed Potato Salad

Some of the cooked potatoes are mashed and blended into the dressing for this chunky potato salad.

4 large baking potatoes (8 ounces each), well washed
⅓ cup white wine vinegar
3 tablespoons light mayonnaise
¼ teaspoon pepper
3 tablespoons pickle relish

1 With a fork, prick the potatoes in several places. Microwave the potatoes according to your oven instructions. Let the potatoes stand for at least 1 minute.

2 Meanwhile, in a large bowl, stir together the vinegar, mayonnaise, and pepper.

3 When cool enough to handle, cut the potatoes into bite-size chunks. Place 1 cup of the potatoes in the bowl with the vinegar-mayonnaise mixture and mash with a potato masher. Stir in the pickle relish.

4 Add the remaining potato chunks and stir to coat. *Makes 6 servings*

Smashed Sweet Potato Salad Substitute sweet potatoes for the baking potatoes. Substitute cider vinegar for the white vinegar and orange marmalade for the pickle relish.

KITCHEN tip

If you don't have a microwave oven, bake the potatoes in a conventional oven at 450°F for 45 to 50 minutes, or until fork-tender.

F.Y.I.

Aromatic rice is an umbrella term for rices that have a toasty, nutty fragrance and a flavor reminiscent of popcorn or roasted nuts. They are primarily long-grain varieties. Perhaps the two best-known aromatic rices are basmati and jasmine, from India and Southeast Asia. They both have a nutlike fragrance while cooking and a delicate, almost buttery flavor. There are also a number of basmati- or jasmine-like aromatic rices that have been developed in this country and that are sold under trade names, including: Jasmati, Kasmati, and Texmati.

Aromatic Rice with Lentils & Black-Eyed Peas

Aromatic rices, such as basmati and jasmine, add dimension to simple bean and rice dishes, but you could certainly substitute regular long-grain white rice in this recipe.

4 cups water
1 cup lentils, picked over and rinsed
1 cup shredded carrots
2 teaspoons minced garlic
¾ teaspoon salt
½ teaspoon rosemary, minced
½ teaspoon pepper
1 cup frozen black-eyed peas
¾ cup basmati or jasmine rice
1 tablespoon olive oil

1 In a large saucepan, bring the water to a boil over high heat. Add the lentils, carrots, garlic, salt, rosemary, and pepper. Return to a boil and boil for 5 minutes.

2 Add the black-eyed peas, rice, and oil. Reduce the heat to a simmer, cover, and cook until both the lentils and rice are tender, 17 to 20 minutes. ***Makes 6 servings***

F.Y.I.

Cremini (crimini) mushrooms are actually a variety of button mushroom with a more intense flavor and a brown-skinned cap. Mature, full-grown cremini are marketed as portobellos. Although cremini are occasionally labeled brown mushrooms or Italian mushrooms, they are now more often labeled baby portobellos, or baby bellas.

Barley, Mushrooms & Peas

Barley and mushrooms are natural companions (and both supply a good amount of soluble fiber). Add green peas to the mix, and you have a really satisfying grain and vegetable side dish.

    2 teaspoons olive oil
    1 cup chopped onion
    2 cups sliced cremini mushrooms
    1 cup quick-cooking barley
    2 cups water
    ¾ teaspoon salt
    ½ teaspoon thyme
    1 cup frozen peas

1 In a medium nonstick saucepan, heat the oil over low heat. Add the onion and cook, stirring occasionally, until the onion is tender, about 7 minutes.

2 Stir in the mushrooms, barley, water, salt, and thyme, and bring to a boil. Reduce to a simmer, cover, and cook until the barley is tender, about 10 minutes.

3 Stir in the peas and cook until heated through, about 3 minutes. Drain any liquid remaining in the pan before serving. *Makes 4 servings*

Mixed Rice Pilaf with Walnuts

Since wild rice is expensive, we've used only a modest amount in this pilaf, but you could use half brown rice and half wild rice. And if you can't find carrot juice—which gives the pilaf a rich golden color, lots of beta carotene, and just a hint of sweetness—use tomato-vegetable juice instead.

per serving	
calories	182
total fat	5.2g
saturated fat	0.8g
cholesterol	0mg
dietary fiber	2g
carbohydrate	30g
protein	5g
sodium	459mg

good source of: beta carotene, vitamin B$_6$

2 teaspoons olive oil
1 cup chopped onions
2 teaspoons minced garlic
¾ cup brown rice
¼ cup wild rice
1½ cups chicken broth
1 cup carrot juice
½ teaspoon salt
¼ teaspoon pepper
¼ cup chopped walnuts

1   In a large nonstick saucepan, heat the oil over low heat. Add the onions and garlic, and cook, stirring occasionally, until the onion is tender, about 7 minutes.

2   Add the brown rice and wild rice, and stir to coat. Add the broth, carrot juice, salt, and pepper, and bring to a boil. Reduce to a simmer, cover, and cook, stirring occasionally, until the rice is tender, about 45 minutes. Stir in the walnuts and serve. ***Makes 6 servings***

Carrot & Raisin Couscous

Couscous is the fastest pasta you can make: The type of couscous available in supermarkets has been precooked, so just needs to be steeped. You just boil some water (in this case, water that's seasoned with garlic, salt, and coriander), stir in the couscous, remove it from the stove, and let it sit for 5 minutes. That's all it takes.

2 cups water
2 teaspoons minced garlic
1 teaspoon paprika
1 teaspoon coriander
¾ teaspoon salt
1 box (10 ounces) couscous
1 cup shredded carrots
⅓ cup raisins
3 tablespoons sliced almonds
2 teaspoons olive oil

1 In a large saucepan, combine the water, garlic, paprika, coriander, and salt. Bring to a boil over medium heat.

2 Stir in the couscous, carrots, and raisins. Cover, remove from the heat, and let stand for 5 minutes or until the couscous has absorbed the liquid.

3 Add the almonds and oil and fluff with a fork. *Makes 8 servings*

Toasted Walnut & Cranberry Couscous Substitute dried cranberries for the raisins, walnuts pieces for the almonds, and walnut oil for the olive oil.

per serving	
calories	185
total fat	2.7g
saturated fat	0.3g
cholesterol	0mg
dietary fiber	3g
carbohydrate	35g
protein	5g
sodium	228mg

good source of: beta carotene, vitamin E

F.Y.I.

Couscous is a tiny pasta used in North African cuisine to make a dish of the same name. Couscous is made of semolina, which is coarsely ground durum wheat. Durum wheat is a high-gluten wheat that is used to make high-quality pastas, because the gluten gives the pasta chewiness and elasticity.

Baked Parmesan Rice & Squash

The flavors in this dish are inspired by an Italian tortellini filling made with pumpkin puree blended with Parmesan and almond macaroon crumbs. In this recipe, winter squash puree takes the place of pumpkin, but the Parmesan and sweet almond flavors are still here.

per serving	
calories	182
total fat	2g
saturated fat	1.1g
cholesterol	4mg
dietary fiber	2g
carbohydrate	36g
protein	6g
sodium	397mg

good source of: beta carotene, folate, thiamin

½ cup chopped onion
2¾ cups water
1 cup rice
¾ teaspoon salt
¾ teaspoon pepper
½ teaspoon rubbed sage
1 package (12 ounces) frozen winter squash puree, thawed
⅓ cup grated Parmesan cheese
2 teaspoons light brown sugar
⅛ teaspoon almond extract

1 Preheat the oven to 350°F. In a Dutch oven or flameproof casserole, heat the onion and ½ cup of the water over medium heat. Cook, stirring occasionally, until the onion is tender, about 5 minutes.

2 Stir in the rice, the remaining 2¼ cups water, the salt, ½ teaspoon of the pepper, and the sage, and bring to a boil. Add the squash puree, half of the Parmesan, the brown sugar, and almond extract, and stir to combine. Cover, place in the oven, and bake for 20 minutes, or until the rice is tender.

3 Stir in the remaining Parmesan and ¼ teaspoon pepper. *Makes 6 servings*

Tex-Mex Cracked Wheat Salad

Bulgur (which is cracked wheat that's been precooked with steam) is usually used to make a Middle Eastern salad called tabbouleh. Here, it's the basis of a salad that includes corn, black beans, and smoky chipotle pepper sauce, giving it a distinctly New World slant. This hearty side dish could easily be converted to a main dish with the addition of 2 cups shredded cooked chicken or cooked shrimp, or 8 ounces of shredded fat-free mozzarella.

1 cup bulgur
2 cups boiling water
¼ cup lime juice
2 tablespoons olive oil
2 teaspoons chipotle pepper sauce
¾ teaspoon oregano
½ teaspoon salt
1 can (15 ounces) black beans, rinsed and drained
1 can (14½ ounces) diced tomatoes
1 cup frozen corn kernels, thawed

1 In a medium heatproof bowl, combine the bulgur and boiling water. Let stand until the bulgur has softened, about 30 minutes. Drain and squeeze dry.

2 In a large bowl, combine the lime juice, oil, chipotle pepper sauce, oregano, and salt. Add the bulgur, beans, tomatoes and their liquid, and the corn, and stir with a fork to combine.

3 Cover and refrigerate at least 1 hour before serving for the flavors to blend. Serve chilled or at room temperature. **_Makes 6 servings_**

per serving	
calories	209
total fat	5.3g
saturated fat	0.8g
cholesterol	0mg
dietary fiber	9g
carbohydrate	36g
protein	8g
sodium	467mg

good source of: fiber, folate, magnesium, potassium, thiamin, vitamin C

F.Y.I.

Also known as smoked jalapeños, chipotles are medium-hot chili peppers with a deep, smoky flavor. They are most typically sold as canned whole chili peppers packed in adobo sauce. There is also a type of bottled hot sauce on the market that is made from chipotles.

Lentil & Pasta Salad with Chunky Tomato Vinaigrette

Canned diced tomatoes come in a range of seasonings, so you could easily switch gears in this recipe and substitute another type of canned tomato, such as Mexican-style.

3 cups water
¾ cup lentils, picked over and rinsed
¾ teaspoon salt
½ teaspoon rubbed sage
⅓ cup ditalini or elbow macaroni
I cup shredded carrots
¼ cup red wine vinegar
I tablespoon olive oil
I can (14½ ounces) diced tomatoes with basil

1 In a large saucepan, bring the water to a boil over high heat. Add the lentils, salt, and sage, and cook for 15 minutes.

2 Add the pasta and carrots, and cook until the lentils and pasta are tender, about 10 minutes. Drain any remaining liquid.

3 Meanwhile, in a large bowl, whisk together the vinegar and oil. Stir in the tomatoes.

4 Add the drained lentil-pasta mixture and toss to combine. Serve warm.
Makes 6 servings

per serving	
calories	146
total fat	2.7g
saturated fat	0.4g
cholesterol	0mg
dietary fiber	9g
carbohydrate	23g
protein	8g
sodium	418mg

good source of: beta carotene, fiber, folate, thiamin, vitamin B$_6$, vitamin C

F.Y.I.

Ever-popular tomatoes supply fiber, thiamin, vitamin B$_6$, iron, potassium, and lots of vitamin C: One medium tomato will give you 66% of the RDA for vitamin C. Tomatoes—especially cooked, condensed forms such as tomato paste, juice, sauce, ketchup, and puree—are an important source of lycopene, a carotenoid with disease-fighting potential. Your body will absorb more lycopene when the tomatoes are cooked with a little fat such as olive oil.

Ranch-Style Rice & Pea Salad

per serving	
calories	202
total fat	1.7g
saturated fat	0.2g
cholesterol	0mg
dietary fiber	6g
carbohydrate	39g
protein	7g
sodium	473mg

good source of: fiber, selenium, vitamin C

Turn this rice salad into a main dish by adding about 2 cups (10 ounces) shredded cooked chicken or turkey, or ¾ pound cooked shrimp. Or for a vegetarian main dish, toss in cubes of one of the flavored baked tofus available in health-food stores and some supermarkets.

⅔ cup brown or white rice
1 can (14½ ounces) diced tomatoes, drained
1 can (15½ ounces) chick-peas, rinsed and drained
1 cup frozen peas, thawed
½ cup fat-free ranch-style salad dressing

1 In a medium saucepan, cook the rice according to package directions. Transfer to a large bowl and fluff to help it cool to room temperature.

2 Add the tomatoes, chick-peas, and green peas. Add the salad dressing and stir to combine. Serve at room temperature or chilled. ***Makes 6 servings***

Curried Rice & Pea Salad Substitute an aromatic rice (such as basmati, Tex-mati, or jasmine) for the brown rice. Stir 2 teaspoons of curry powder into the ranch-style dressing.

Dilled Green Bean & Mushroom Salad

Canned sliced water chestnuts are a quick way to add a bit of heft as well as crunch to a vegetable salad.

1 pound green beans
½ cup fat-free honey-mustard dressing
⅓ cup snipped fresh dill
¼ teaspoon pepper
2 cups sliced mushrooms
½ cup canned sliced water chestnuts, drained

1 In a vegetable steamer, cook the green beans until crisp-tender, 5 to 7 minutes. Rinse under cold water and drain well.

2 Meanwhile, in a large bowl, combine the honey-mustard dressing, dill, and pepper.

3 Add the warm green beans, mushrooms, and water chestnuts, and toss to combine. Serve at room temperature or chilled. *Makes 4 servings*

per serving	
calories	95
total fat	0.3g
saturated fat	0g
cholesterol	0mg
dietary fiber	6g
carbohydrate	22g
protein	3g
sodium	132mg

good source of: fiber, folate, potassium, vitamin C

KITCHEN *tip*

One of the best ways to "mince" the feathery fronds of fresh dill is to use a pair of scissors. Hold the dill sprigs over a bowl and snip the herb into tiny pieces.

per serving	
calories	115
total fat	3.4g
saturated fat	1.4g
cholesterol	5mg
dietary fiber	5g
carbohydrate	18g
protein	5g
sodium	510mg

good source of: beta carotene, fiber, folate, potassium, riboflavin, thiamin, vitamin C, vitamin E

F.Y.I.

A rich source of antioxidants, blueberries are low in calories and rich in flavor. Blueberries also contain significant amounts of vitamin C, as well as pectin, a soluble fiber that helps lower cholesterol levels.

Red, White & Blueberry Salad

Tomatoes (which are technically a fruit) have a slight sweetness to them that marries well with the berries in this savory side salad. Grape tomatoes are especially sweet, but if you can't find them, use small cherry tomatoes instead.

⅓ cup fat-free balsamic dressing
1 tablespoon honey-mustard
¼ teaspoon pepper
8 cups mixed salad greens
1 cup raspberries
1 cup blueberries
1 cup grape tomatoes
½ cup crumbled reduced-fat feta cheese

1 In a small bowl, stir together the balsamic dressing, honey-mustard, and pepper.

2 Arrange the greens on 4 salad plates. Top with the raspberries, blueberries, tomatoes, and feta. Drizzle the dressing on top. ***Makes 4 servings***

Black Bean & Cabbage Salad

Tomato-vegetable juice has enough texture to be the basis for an easy low-fat salad dressing. For an extra kick, try the spicy version of tomato-vegetable juice in the dressing.

> ½ cup tomato-vegetable juice
> 2 tablespoons red wine vinegar
> 2 teaspoons olive oil
> ¼ teaspoon salt
> ¼ teaspoon pepper
> 1 can (15½ ounces) black beans, rinsed and drained
> 2 cups packaged coleslaw mixture
> 1 cup chopped green bell pepper

1 In a large bowl, stir together the tomato-vegetable juice, vinegar, oil, salt, and pepper.

2 Add the beans, coleslaw mixture, and bell pepper, and toss to combine. *Makes 4 servings*

Turkey, White Bean & Cabbage Salad For a main-dish salad, substitute white wine vinegar for the red wine vinegar and add ½ teaspoon tarragon to the dressing in step 1. Substitute cannellini beans for the black beans. Add 2 cups (10 ounces) shredded roast turkey breast to the salad in step 2.

per serving	
calories	116
total fat	3g
saturated fat	0.4g
cholesterol	0mg
dietary fiber	4g
carbohydrate	19g
protein	5g
sodium	542mg

good source of: fiber, folate, thiamin, vitamin C

Pea, Water Chestnut & Roasted Pepper Salad

Water chestnuts are usually relegated to Chinese stir-fries, but they add welcome crunch to salads.

> 3 tablespoons balsamic vinegar
> 2 teaspoons olive oil
> 2 teaspoons Dijon mustard
> 1 teaspoon sugar
> ½ teaspoon salt
> 1 package (10 ounces) frozen peas, thawed
> 1 can (8 ounces) sliced water chestnuts, drained
> ½ cup jarred roasted red peppers, sliced

1 In a serving bowl, combine the vinegar, oil, mustard, sugar, and salt.

2 Add the peas, water chestnuts, and roasted peppers. Toss to combine. Serve at room temperature or chilled. ***Makes 4 servings***

Pasta Salad with Peas & Water Chestnuts Cook 8 ounces of penne or fusilli pasta according to package directions. Drain. Make a triple batch of the dressing in step 1, but use only ½ teaspoon of salt. Toss the warm pasta with the dressing and the remaining salad ingredients.

Moroccan Carrot Slaw

Ground cumin and coriander lend an exotic note to the creamy dressing for this slaw. In addition to being a delicious side salad, it makes a great topping for burgers and other sandwiches.

⅔ cup plain fat-free yogurt
¼ cup lemon juice
1 tablespoon light mayonnaise
1 tablespoon sugar
1 teaspoon paprika
¾ teaspoon cumin
¾ teaspoon coriander
½ teaspoon salt
1 bag (10 ounces) shredded carrots

1 In a large bowl, stir together the yogurt, lemon juice, mayonnaise, sugar, paprika, cumin, coriander, and salt.

2 Add the carrots and toss to coat. Serve at room temperature or chilled. *Makes 4 servings*

ON THE *Menu*

This mildly spiced carrot slaw would be a nice side dish for Apricot-Glazed Roast Pork (*page 57*), along with a baked potato. For dessert, serve Sweet Cheese Pie (*page 125*).

Off-the-Shelf

Basically just a crustless pumpkin pie, this delicious baked pudding takes advantage of some off-the-shelf ingredients: canned pumpkin pie mix and refrigerated egg substitute. Once the ingredients are assembled (there are only four of them!), it should take only 5 minutes to put the pudding together. The rest is unattended cooking in the oven. Serve the hot pudding with a dollop of lightly sweetened fat-free sour cream or a scoop of low-fat vanilla frozen yogurt.

Baked Pumpkin Pudding

1 can (15 ounces) pumpkin pie mix
1 cup low-fat (1%) milk
½ cup egg substitute or 4 large egg whites
¼ cup raisins

1 Preheat the oven to 350°F.

2 In a medium bowl, stir together the pumpkin pie mix, milk, egg substitute, and raisins.

3 Pour the pumpkin mixture into an 8-inch square glass baking dish. Bake for 40 minutes, or until the pudding is lightly browned and set in the center. *Makes 6 servings*

PER SERVING 114 calories, 0.6g total fat (0.3g saturated), 2mg cholesterol, 6g dietary fiber, 26g carbohydrate, 4g protein, 187mg sodium
Good source of: **beta carotene, fiber**

Sweet Cheese Pie

This is similar to an Italian-style cheesecake, but it's baked in a distinctly American graham cracker crust. If you prefer, substitute orange juice for the Marsala.

½ cup raisins
3 tablespoons Marsala or dark rum
1¼ cups low-fat cottage cheese
½ cup part-skim ricotta cheese
⅔ cup sugar
3 tablespoons flour
½ cup egg substitute or 4 large egg whites
¾ teaspoon vanilla extract
1 reduced-fat prebaked 9-inch graham cracker crust

1 Preheat the oven to 325°F.

2 In a small bowl, combine the raisins and Marsala and set aside.

3 In a food processor, combine the cottage cheese, ricotta, sugar, flour, egg substitute, and vanilla, and puree. Stir in the raisins and Marsala.

4 Place the crust on a baking sheet. Pour the cheese mixture into the crust and bake for 50 minutes, or until the edges are starting to brown and the center is firm.

5 Turn the oven off and leave the pie inside with the door closed for 1 hour. Cool completely on a wire rack. Serve at room temperature or chilled.
Makes 8 wedges

Crumb-Topped Baked Pineapple

This baked pineapple dessert is similar to a brown betty, a dish that dates back to Colonial times.

1 cup graham cracker crumbs
⅓ cup packed light brown sugar
¼ cup walnut pieces
½ teaspoon cinnamon
¼ teaspoon salt
1 tablespoon extra-light olive oil
2 cans (20 ounces each) juice-packed crushed pineapple, drained
¼ cup seedless raspberry jam

1 Preheat the oven to 350°F. In a food processor, combine the graham cracker crumbs, brown sugar, walnuts, cinnamon, and salt, and pulse until the nuts are finely ground. Add the oil and pulse until the crumb mixture is evenly moistened.

2 In an 8-inch square glass baking dish, stir together the pineapple and the raspberry jam. Scatter the crumbs on top and bake for 30 minutes, or until the pineapple is piping hot and the crumbs are crusty. *Makes 4 servings*

Sweet Cherry Sundaes

Be sure to let the frozen yogurt stand in the refrigerator for about 30 minutes before serving so it will be soft enough to scoop. To bring out the flavor in the almonds, toast them for about 5 minutes in a toaster oven.

2 cups frozen pitted sweet cherries, thawed
½ cup raspberry all-fruit spread
1 tablespoon balsamic vinegar
2 teaspoons cornstarch blended with 1 tablespoon water
⅛ teaspoon almond extract
1 pint vanilla low-fat frozen yogurt
2 tablespoons sliced almonds

1 In a medium saucepan, combine the cherries, fruit spread, vinegar, and cornstarch mixture. Bring to a simmer over medium heat. Cook, stirring, until slightly thickened, about 1 minute.

2 Remove from the heat and stir in the almond extract. Let the cherry sauce cool to room temperature.

3 Serve the frozen yogurt topped with the cherry sauce and the almonds.
Makes 4 servings

F.Y.I.

Low in calories (½ cup has only 52) and bursting with flavor, cherries contain soluble fiber and vitamin C as well as phytochemicals. Proponents of a folk remedy for gout believe that drinking cherry juice can help relieve pain and inflammation linked to gout, though there is no scientific evidence to support this belief.

Off-the-Shelf

Angel food cake is a naturally fat-free dessert. It is made with just egg whites, sugar, and flour, and not a speck of fat. However, it is also time-consuming to make from scratch, since it involves beating about one dozen egg whites. Luckily, storebought angel food cake makes a good off-the-shelf dessert. Just doctor up some chocolate syrup (which is virtually fat free) with some espresso powder and cinnamon, and drizzle the sauce over slices of angel food cake that have been toasted under the broiler.

Orange-Broiled Angel Food Cake with Mocha Sauce

1 cup chocolate syrup
2 teaspoons instant espresso powder
½ teaspoon cinnamon
¼ cup orange all-fruit spread
1 tablespoon lemon juice
1 storebought angel food cake (11 ounces), cut into 8 slices

1 Preheat the broiler.

2 In a medium bowl, stir together the chocolate syrup, espresso powder, and cinnamon until well combined.

3 In a small bowl, combine the fruit spread and the lemon juice.

4 Place the cake slices on a broiler pan and brush with the fruit spread mixture. Broil 4 to 6 inches from the heat for 1 minute or until lightly toasted. Serve the cake drizzled with the mocha sauce. ***Makes 8 servings***

PER SLICE 196 calories, 0.5g total fat (0.2g saturated), 0mg cholesterol, 1g dietary fiber, 48g carbohydrate, 3g protein, 236mg sodium

Baked Bananas

Delicious just as they are, these baked bananas could be converted into a banana split by topping them with a scoop of low-fat frozen yogurt and a sprinkling of toasted almonds or walnuts.

per serving	
calories	176
total fat	0.6g
saturated fat	0.3g
cholesterol	0mg
dietary fiber	3g
carbohydrate	45g
protein	1g
sodium	10mg

good source of: potassium, vitamin B$_6$

$\frac{1}{3}$ cup packed light brown sugar
3 tablespoons lime juice
$\frac{1}{4}$ teaspoon nutmeg
4 bananas (1 pound) peeled

1 Preheat the oven to 350°F. In a 7 x 11-inch glass or ceramic baking dish, stir together the brown sugar, lime juice, and nutmeg.

2 Add the bananas, turning them to coat with the brown sugar mixture. Place in the oven and bake for 10 minutes.

3 Turn the bananas over and bake for 7 minutes longer, or until tender. Serve the bananas warm, with the sauce spooned on top. *Makes 4 servings*

Maple Baked Bananas Use maple syrup instead of brown sugar and lemon juice instead of lime juice.

Fallen Mocha Soufflé Cake

Serve wedges of this delicious, dense (and low-calorie!!) espresso-flavored chocolate cake with a scoop of low-fat coffee frozen yogurt. If you'd like to really gild the lily, drizzle the yogurt with a little bit of chocolate sauce.

per wedge	
calories	102
total fat	1g
saturated fat	0.5g
cholesterol	18mg
dietary fiber	1g
carbohydrate	22g
protein	3g
sodium	79mg

good source of:
selenium

¾ cup sugar
½ cup unsweetened cocoa powder
¼ cup chocolate syrup
1½ teaspoons instant espresso powder
½ teaspoon vanilla extract
1 large egg, separated
½ cup flour
4 large egg whites
¼ teaspoon salt
¼ teaspoon cream of tartar

1 Preheat the oven to 375°F. Line the bottom of a 9-inch springform pan with wax paper. Spray the paper and the sides of the pan with nonstick cooking spray.

2 In a medium bowl, combine ½ cup of the sugar, the cocoa, chocolate syrup, espresso powder, and vanilla, and stir until smooth. Stir in the egg yolk and flour.

3 In a medium bowl, with an electric mixer, beat the 5 egg whites and salt until frothy. Add the cream of tartar and beat to soft peaks. Gradually add the remaining ¼ cup sugar, 1 tablespoon at a time, until stiff peaks form.

4 Stir one-fourth of the egg whites into the chocolate mixture to lighten it, then fold the chocolate mixture into the remaining egg whites until just combined. Pour the batter into the springform.

5 Bake for 25 minutes, or until a cake tester inserted in the center comes out clean. Cool in the pan on a rack. Remove the sides of the pan and cut the cake into 12 wedges. *Makes 12 wedges*

Off-the-Shelf

Lazy Lime Pie

Anyone who has ever **made a real** Key lime pie knows that it involves crushing graham crackers for a crust and making an egg-based custard for the filling. Our off-the-shelf solution is to use lime gelatin as a thickener and a storebought reduced-fat graham cracker crust. In addition, we've cut some fat out by using low-fat evaporated milk instead of the full-fat sweetened condensed milk called for in a traditional Key lime pie. The lime juice called for is just regular lime juice, but if you know where you can get a bottle of real Key lime juice, use it instead.

1 package (3 ounces) lime-flavored gelatin dessert
½ cup boiling water
½ cup lime juice
1 can (12 ounces) evaporated low-fat (2%) milk
1 reduced-fat prebaked 9-inch graham cracker crust

1 In a large heatproof bowl, combine the lime gelatin with the boiling water, stirring until dissolved.

2 Stir in the lime juice and evaporated milk until well blended. Pour the mixture into the crust and refrigerate until set, at least 2 hours. ***Makes 6 servings***

PER SERVING 189 calories, 4.2g total fat (1.2g saturated), 5mg cholesterol, 0g dietary fiber, 32g carbohydrate, 7g protein, 184mg sodium
Good source of: calcium, riboflavin

Fresh Blueberry Granola Crisp

per serving	
calories	198
total fat	1.6g
saturated fat	0.4g
cholesterol	0mg
dietary fiber	4g
carbohydrate	46g
protein	3g
sodium	153mg

good source of: folate, niacin, riboflavin, thiamin, vitamin B_{12}, vitamin E

For the topping on this quickly assembled dessert, you could use any low-fat granola, such as those sold in bulk in health-food stores. But we tested this with a national brand of granola available in supermarkets and it worked very nicely. For an extra treat, serve the crisp with a scoop of frozen yogurt or a dollop of lightly sweetened reduced-fat sour cream.

> 2 pints blueberries
> ¼ cup flour
> ¼ teaspoon allspice
> ¼ teaspoon salt
> ⅓ cup sugar
> 1½ cups low-fat granola

1 Preheat the oven to 350°F. In a small bowl, stir together the blueberries, flour, allspice, and salt.

2 Transfer the berries to a 9-inch pie plate. Sprinkle the sugar over the berries and scatter the granola over the top.

3 Bake for 30 minutes, or until the fruit is thick and bubbling. Serve warm or at room temperature. ***Makes 6 servings***

Three-Berry Granola Crisp Reduce the blueberries to 1 pint and add ½ pint each raspberries and strawberries. Add ½ teaspoon cinnamon and ⅛ teaspoon ground cloves (in addition to the allspice) to the berries in step 1.

F.Y.I.

Along with supplying fiber, the blueberries and the granola supply a good amount of folate in this baked blueberry crisp. While folate occurs naturally in the blueberries, the granola has been fortified with this important B vitamin, which is called "folic acid" when it is added to a food or supplement.

Easy Rice Pudding

per serving	
calories	233
total fat	1.7g
saturated fat	1.1g
cholesterol	6mg
dietary fiber	1g
carbohydrate	48g
protein	5g
sodium	137mg

Here's a simple, low-cholesterol rice pudding. It's an ideal use for leftover rice, but if you don't happen to have any, cook 1 cup of rice according to package directions to yield 3 cups cooked.

1½ cups low-fat (1%) milk
½ cup sugar
¾ teaspoon cinnamon
¼ teaspoon salt
3 cups cooked rice
⅓ cup dried cherries, dried cranberries, or raisins
¼ cup reduced-fat sour cream

1 In a medium saucepan, stir together the milk, sugar, cinnamon, and salt. Bring to a simmer over medium heat.

2 Stir in the cooked rice. Return to a simmer, cover, and cook until the rice is creamy, about 10 minutes. Remove from the heat and stir in the dried cherries.

3 Let cool to room temperature. Stir in the sour cream and refrigerate until chilled. ***Makes 6 servings***

Plum-Ginger Rice Pudding Substitute ground ginger for the cinnamon. Use diced dried plums (prunes) instead of dried cherries. Add ½ teaspoon vanilla when stirring in the fruit in step 2.

Off-the-Shelf

Clafouti is a traditional home-style French dessert made with a batter that closely resembles pancake batter—which is why we based this recipe on a storebought baking mix intended for pancakes. Since most such baking mixes are pretty high in fat, we used a reduced-fat version. You could also make this dessert with other fruit: Try a combination of 1 cup cherries and 1 cup peach slices. Add ½ teaspoon cinnamon to the fruit (in addition to the nutmeg).

Cherry Clafouti

2 cups frozen pitted sweet cherries, thawed
2 tablespoons plus ¼ cup sugar
½ teaspoon nutmeg
1 cup reduced-fat all-purpose baking mix
½ cup plain fat-free yogurt
¼ cup fat-free milk
¼ cup egg substitute or 2 egg whites
1 teaspoon vanilla extract

1 Preheat the oven to 350°F. Place the cherries in a 9-inch pie plate. Sprinkle 2 tablespoons of the sugar and ¼ teaspoon of the nutmeg over the cherries.

2 In a medium bowl, stir together the remaining ¼ cup sugar, the remaining ¼ teaspoon nutmeg, the baking mix, yogurt, milk, egg substitute, and vanilla until smooth. Spoon the batter over the fruit.

3 Bake for 40 minutes, or until the cake is richly browned and a toothpick inserted in the center comes out clean. ***Makes 6 servings***

PER SERVING 181 calories, 2g total fat (0.5g saturated), 1mg cholesterol, 2g dietary fiber, 36g carbohydrate, 5g protein, 272mg sodium

Tropical Fruit Compote

per serving	
calories	227
total fat	1.3g
saturated fat	0.1g
cholesterol	0mg
dietary fiber	3g
carbohydrate	54g
protein	2g
sodium	71mg

good source of:
vitamin C

Served on its own or topped with a dollop of reduced-fat sour cream or fat-free yogurt, fruit compote makes a wonderful dessert. But why stop there? Use it as an accompaniment to meat or poultry. Stir it into a bowl of hot cereal or a cup of yogurt or cottage cheese. Spread it on your morning toast as is, or stir a spoonful into reduced-fat cream cheese and spread on a bagel.

1 can (11½ ounces) mango nectar
¼ cup water
¼ teaspoon allspice
¼ teaspoon pepper
⅛ teaspoon salt
1 package (7 ounces) dried tropical fruit mix (about 1 cup)
1 package (6 ounces) dried pineapple
2 tablespoons lime juice
½ teaspoon vanilla extract

1 In a medium nonaluminum saucepan, bring the nectar, water, allspice, pepper, and salt to a boil over medium heat. Add the fruit and reduce to a simmer.

2 Cook, uncovered, until the fruit is tender and the liquid is syrupy, about 15 minutes. Cool to room temperature and stir in the lime juice and vanilla. Serve at room temperature or chilled. *Makes 6 servings*

Peach & Apricot Compote Substitute 1½ cups peach nectar for the mango nectar. Omit the allspice and add ½ teaspoon ground ginger. Use 1 cup dried peaches and 1 cup dried apricots instead of the tropical fruit and pineapple.

Plum & Pear Compote Substitute 1½ cups grape juice for the mango nectar. Add 2 tablespoons of sugar to the juice when heating it in step 1. Use 1 cup pitted dried plums (prunes) and 1 cup dried pears instead of the tropical fruit and pineapple. Substitute orange juice for the lime juice in step 2.

Peaches & Cream

This is a good trick for an easy dessert, though you have to think about it ahead of time because it takes 2 hours to chill. The rest is a snap, and you can make it with all sorts of fruit, or even storebought applesauce. You just need about 2 cups of fruit puree.

1 envelope unflavored gelatin
¼ cup water
1 package (20 ounces) frozen peach slices, thawed
⅓ cup packed light brown sugar
3 tablespoons lemon juice
⅛ teaspoon almond extract
½ cup plain fat-free yogurt
¼ cup reduced-fat sour cream

1 In a small, heatproof bowl, sprinkle the gelatin over the water and let stand until softened, about 2 minutes. Set the bowl in a pan of simmering water and heat until the gelatin dissolves, about 3 minutes. Set aside to cool to room temperature.

2 In a food processor, puree the gelatin mixture, peaches, brown sugar, lemon juice, and almond extract until smooth.

3 Transfer the puree to a large bowl. Stir in the yogurt and sour cream until blended. Spoon into a serving bowl, 4 individual bowls, or 4 wineglasses, and refrigerate until set, about 2 hours. ***Makes 4 servings***

Apricot-Rum Sundaes

This is a nearly instant dessert. It probably will take more time to bring the frozen yogurt to scooping consistency than it will to make the apricot-rum sauce for these sundaes.

per serving	
calories	190
total fat	3g
saturated fat	1g
cholesterol	5mg
dietary fiber	2g
carbohydrate	34g
protein	6g
sodium	67mg

good source of: calcium, riboflavin, vitamin B$_{12}$

1 can (15½ ounces) water-packed apricot halves, drained
2 tablespoons light brown sugar
4 teaspoons dark rum or orange juice
1 tablespoon orange all-fruit spread
⅛ teaspoon allspice
1 pint frozen low-fat vanilla yogurt
2 tablespoons sliced almonds

1 In a food processor, puree the apricots, brown sugar, rum, fruit spread, and allspice.

2 Spoon the apricot sauce over the frozen yogurt and sprinkle the sliced almonds on top. *Makes 4 servings*

Plum-Brandy Sundaes Substitute canned plums for the apricot halves, brandy or orange liqueur for the rum, and apricot fruit spread for the orange.

F.Y.I.

Although you'll get the most vitamin C from apricots by eating them raw, other substances—such as beta carotene and the soluble fiber pectin— are actually made more available to the body when the apricots are cooked.

Storebought pound cake mix makes a convenient topping for cranberries and pineapple in this quick-to-assemble upside-down cake. Pound cake gets its name from the ingredients in a traditional recipe: a pound of sugar, a pound of flour, a pound of eggs, and a pound of butter. Luckily, this reduced-fat mix rescues the cake from the 100 grams of fat in the original recipe.

Cranberry-Pineapple Upside-Down Cake

1 can (16 ounces) whole-berry cranberry sauce
1 can (8 ounces) juice-packed crushed pineapple, undrained
½ teaspoon ground ginger
1 package (16 ounces) low-fat pound cake mix
¾ cup fat-free milk
⅓ cup egg substitute or 3 large egg whites

1 Preheat the oven to 350°F. In a 9-inch square glass baking dish, stir together the cranberry sauce, pineapple, and ginger.

2 In a large bowl, combine the cake mix, milk, and egg substitute, and beat according to package directions. Pour the batter over the cranberry mixture.

3 Bake for 45 minutes, or until the cake is golden brown and a toothpick inserted in the center of the cake comes out clean. Cool to room temperature and serve from the pan, cutting the cake into squares. *Makes 9 squares*

PER SQUARE 322 calories, 6.4g total fat (1.6g saturated), 1mg cholesterol, 1g dietary fiber, 62g carbohydrate, 4g protein, 229mg sodium

F.Y.I.

When you cook the apples for applesauce, a type of soluble fiber called pectin is released when the apples' cell walls soften as they are heated. Like other types of soluble fiber, pectin helps to lower cholesterol. And it may also be useful for weight control. Pectin forms a viscous gel in the intestines, which slows the emptying of the stomach and creates a feeling of fullness. Pectin is used commercially as a binding and thickening agent in jams, jellies, and preserves.

Breakfast Bread Pudding with Apple-Raspberry Sauce

For a real treat, you could serve the bread pudding topped with some fresh raspberries and a dusting of confectioners' sugar.

2½ cups low-fat (1%) milk
½ cup egg substitute or 4 large egg whites
¼ cup sugar
½ teaspoon vanilla extract
¼ teaspoon cinnamon
¼ teaspoon salt
8 slices oatmeal bread, toasted and torn into bite-size pieces
1⅓ cups raspberry applesauce or mixed berry applesauce

1 Preheat the oven to 350°F. Spray an 8-inch square baking dish with non-stick cooking spray.

2 In a large bowl, whisk together the milk, egg substitute, sugar, vanilla, cinnamon, and salt.

3 Place the toast in the baking dish and spread the apple-raspberry sauce on top. Pour the milk mixture over the apple-raspberry sauce.

4 Bake for 30 minutes, or until the pudding is set and the top is golden brown and puffed. Serve warm, at room temperature, or chilled. **Makes 6 servings**

Asparagus & Pea Frittata

¾ cup water
1 cup dehydrated hash brown potatoes (from a 6-ounce box)
1 can (10½ ounces) cut asparagus, drained
1 package (10 ounces) frozen peas, thawed
¾ teaspoon salt
½ teaspoon tarragon
2 teaspoons olive oil
1½ cups egg substitute or 12 egg whites
3 tablespoons grated Parmesan

1 In a 10-inch nonstick skillet, combine the water and potatoes. Cook over low heat until the potatoes have softened, about 7 minutes.

2 Add the asparagus and peas to the skillet. Sprinkle the salt and tarragon over the vegetables. Pour the oil down the sides of the pan so that it goes under the vegetables.

3 Pour the egg substitute over the vegetables and sprinkle with the Parmesan. Cook over low heat, without stirring, until the eggs are set around the edges and almost set in the center, about 15 minutes.

4 Cover and cook until the center is set, about 5 minutes. Serve in wedges from the pan. *Makes 4 servings*

PER SERVING **228 calories, 4.6g total fat (1.3g saturated), 4mg cholesterol, 5g dietary fiber, 30g carbohydrate, 16g protein, 805mg sodium**
Good source of: **riboflavin, vitamin C**

Homemade hash brown potatoes are wonderful, but they involve a lot of preparation. You have to grate potatoes on a box grater (or in a food processor), and it's not a simple task, especially if you have any kind of joint pain in the wrist or fingers. A very reasonable alternative is packaged dehydrated hash browns, especially when they are incorporated into a one-pot breakfast dish like a frittata. Frittatas, which are Italian-style omelets, generally use the eggs as a binder for ingredients such as vegetables and meat. In this meatless rendition, hash browns, asparagus, and green peas are cooked in a tarragon-scented egg mixture, topped with Parmesan cheese.

Carrot-Cardamom Tea Bread

Carrots, a touch of orange juice, and the heady aroma of the sweet spice cardamom give this tea bread a mildly exotic flavor. Serve on its own or with orange marmalade and reduced-fat cream cheese.

per slice	
calories	191
total fat	6.2g
saturated fat	0.8g
cholesterol	0mg
dietary fiber	1g
carbohydrate	32g
protein	3g
sodium	216mg

good source of: beta carotene

1½ cups flour
1½ teaspoons cardamom
1 teaspoon ground ginger
½ teaspoon cinnamon
1 teaspoon baking powder
¾ teaspoon baking soda
½ teaspoon salt
1 cup sugar
⅓ cup extra-light olive oil
½ cup egg substitute or 4 large egg whites
¼ cup orange juice
2¼ cups shredded carrots

1 Preheat the oven to 350°F. Generously spray a 9 x 5-inch loaf pan with nonstick cooking spray. In a medium bowl, stir together the flour, cardamom, ginger, cinnamon, baking powder, baking soda, and salt.

2 In another bowl, with an electric mixer, beat the sugar and oil until light and creamy. Beat in the egg substitute until well combined. Beat in the orange juice. Stir in the flour mixture. Fold the carrots into the batter.

3 Pour the batter into the loaf pan. Bake for 55 minutes, or until a toothpick inserted in the center comes out clean. Cool for 10 minutes in the pan on a rack. Then invert onto the wire rack to cool completely. ***Makes 12 slices***

Lemon Poppyseed Tea Bread

The zest of a lemon is the thin, colored layer of peel that contains all of the fragrant oils. When you peel the lemon to get the zest, be sure to take just this thin layer and not the spongy white pith beneath it. The white pith at best has no flavor, and at worst can be bitter.

> 2 lemons
> 1 cup sugar
> 2 tablespoons poppy seeds
> 2 cups flour
> 1 teaspoon baking powder
> ½ teaspoon baking soda
> ½ teaspoon salt
> ⅓ cup extra-light olive oil
> ¼ cup egg substitute or 2 large egg whites
> 1 cup buttermilk

1 Preheat the oven to 350°F. Generously spray a 9 x 5-inch loaf pan with nonstick cooking spray.

2 With a vegetable peeler, peel the zest from the lemons in long strips. In a food processor, combine the strips of lemon zest, ½ cup of the sugar, and the poppy seeds. Process until the lemon zest is finely ground.

3 In a medium bowl, combine the flour, baking powder, baking soda, and salt. Set aside.

4 In another medium bowl, with an electric mixer, beat the remaining ½ cup sugar, the lemon zest-poppyseed mixture, and the oil until well combined. Add the egg substitute in 3 additions, beating well after each.

5 On low speed, alternately beat the flour mixture and the buttermilk into the batter, beginning and ending with the flour mixture.

6 Spoon the batter into the loaf pan and bake for 55 minutes, or until a toothpick inserted in the center comes out clean. Cool for 10 minutes in the pan on a wire rack. Then turn the loaf out onto the rack to cool completely.
Makes 12 slices

F.Y.I.

Olive oil that has little or no olive flavor is labeled "Light," "Extra-light," or "Mild-flavored," depending on the manufacturer. These olive oils are intentionally bland so that you can use them in places where you don't want the oil to add flavor, such as in baked goods or pancakes. The "light" on the label refers to the flavor of the oil and not its fat content, since all olive oils have the same number of calories and fat grams; and all of them have the same high level of heart-healthy monounsaturated fats.

Off-the-Shelf

Corn muffin mix is a good place to start, but there are some tricks you can use to make both its flavor and texture more interesting, and also lower its fat content. Instead of 1 whole egg and ½ cup of whole milk, this cornbread is made with egg substitute and creamed corn. The creamed corn and reduced-fat cheese also makes the bread moister.

Creamy Cornbread

1 box (8½ ounces) corn muffin mix
1 teaspoon chili powder
1 can (14¾ ounces) no-salt-added creamed corn
¼ cup egg substitute or 2 large egg whites
½ cup shredded reduced-fat Cheddar cheese

1 Preheat the oven to 400°F. Spray an 8-inch square baking pan with non-stick cooking spray.

2 Place the corn muffin mix in a large bowl. Stir in the chili powder. Make a well in the center and pour in the creamed corn, egg substitute, and Cheddar. Stir until just combined.

3 Pour the mixture into the pan. Bake for 25 minutes, or until a toothpick inserted in the center comes out clean. Cool in the pan on a wire rack. Cut into squares. *Makes 9 squares*

PER SQUARE 166 calories, 4g total fat (1.5g saturated), 10mg cholesterol, 1g dietary fiber, 28g carbohydrate, 6g protein, 262mg sodium

per serving	
calories	189
total fat	0.8g
saturated fat	0.3g
cholesterol	0mg
dietary fiber	3g
carbohydrate	46g
protein	2g
sodium	3mg

good source of: potassium, vitamin B$_6$, vitamin C

Banana-Tangerine Shake

If you don't have time to sit down to a real breakfast, the next best thing is a breakfast fruit shake. Banana is an especially good ingredient, because it makes the shake thick. With so many interesting fruit juices and fruit juice blends available, you can use the basic proportions here and try this shake with other flavors. For an easy flavor twist, use maple syrup as the sweetener instead of honey. Or use one of the darker honeys available, like buckwheat.

½ cup tangerine juice
1 medium banana, cut into chunks
1 teaspoon honey
½ teaspoon vanilla extract
2 ice cubes

In a blender, combine the tangerine juice, banana, honey, and vanilla. Add the ice and blend until thick and smooth. ***Makes 1 serving***

per serving	
calories	147
total fat	1.5g
saturated fat	0.8g
cholesterol	7mg
dietary fiber	2g
carbohydrate	31g
protein	5g
sodium	132mg

good source of:
calcium, potassium, thiamin, vitamin C

Creamy Strawberry-Pineapple Smoothie

If you aren't a fan of buttermilk, you could make this breakfast smoothie with yogurt instead. The warm spices—allspice and nutmeg—are a perfect match for pineapple.

    1 cup buttermilk
    1 cup canned juice-packed pineapple chunks, drained
    ½ cup frozen strawberries, unthawed
    1 tablespoon honey
    2 teaspoons lime juice
    ⅛ teaspoon allspice
    ⅛ teaspoon nutmeg
    4 ice cubes

In a blender, combine the buttermilk, pineapple, strawberries, honey, lime juice, allspice, nutmeg, and ice cubes, and puree until thick and smooth.
Makes 2 servings

THE SAVVY SHOPPER

all-fruit spread There does not seem to be any consistency in labeling for fruit spreads: they can be called various things, including spreadable fruit, all-fruit, or 100% fruit. But underneath it all they are all "jams" that are made with nothing but fruit and fruit juice and have no refined sugar. They are slightly lower in calories and carbohydrates than regular jam: 1 tablespoon of regular jam has about 50 calories and 13 grams of sugars; 1 tablespoon of all-fruit spread has 40 calories and about 8 grams of sugars.

allspice Allspice is a dark, round, dried berry about the size of a large peppercorn and is available as whole berries or ground. Allspice tastes like a blend of spices (cloves, cinnamon, and nutmeg), and many people mistakenly take its name to mean that it is, in fact, a blend. Like black pepper, allspice has the most flavor if freshly ground when you use it.

beans, canned Many types of beans—black beans, red kidney beans, cannellini (white kidney beans), chick-peas, pinto beans—are available in canned form. They are a great and convenient source of low-fat protein, complex carbohydrates, soluble fiber, and the B vitamin folate. The only downside to them is their sodium content. However, if you place the beans in a strainer and run cold water over them to rinse off the liquid they come packed in, you will reduce the sodium content considerably. This also removes some of the water-soluble B vitamins, but it's a fair trade. Keep canned beans in your pantry, but consider cooking your own beans from scratch and then freezing them so you can use them at a moment's notice.

carrot juice Carrot juice is a much overlooked ingredient. Most people think of it as a "health" drink and not as a cooking ingredient. It is, however, a wonderful substitute for broth in soups, stews, sauces, marinades, and can also be used in baked goods. Its subtle natural sweetness brings out the flavors in savory dishes. It also adds a spectacular amount of the antioxidant beta carotene. Canned carrot juice, available in supermarkets, has the highest concentration of beta carotene. Refrigerated carrot juice, found in supermarkets and health-food stores, is lower in beta carotene, but still a good option.

carrots, baby The bags of "baby" carrots available in supermarkets aren't baby carrots at all. They are actually pieces cut from narrow, straight-sided carrots specially grown to be used this way. The pieces are then processed to remove their skin and round their edges. They not only make a great snack, but they are small enough to throw into soups and stews and cook as is.

cayenne pepper This ground spice—very hot and orange-red or deep red in color—is based on very pungent peppers grown in Louisiana, Africa, India, and Mexico (although it is sometimes made from other type of chili pepper). Some spice companies also offer a ground spice labeled simply "red pepper."

cheese, feta Feta cheese is a soft, crumbly, cured Greek cheese, traditionally made from sheep's or goat's milk. Chalk-white and rindless, feta is usually available as rectangular blocks packed in brine; it's best to rinse it before using to eliminate some of the sodium. Because feta is so highly flavorful, a little goes a long way.

cheese, parmesan Parmesan cheese is an intensely flavored, hard grating cheese. Genuine Italian Parmesan, stamped "Parmigiano-Reggiano" on the rind, is produced in the

Emilia-Romagna region, and tastes richly nutty with a slight sweetness. For the best, freshest flavor, buy Parmesan in blocks and grate it as needed. For a fine, fluffy texture that melts into hot foods, grate the cheese in a hand-cranked grater. However, pregrated Parmesan is a perfectly fine option; it will just have a saltier, less nutty, flavor and will not melt as well.

chick-peas Chick-peas are round, cream-colored legumes that are used extensively in cuisines ranging from the Middle East to Latin America (where they are called garbanzos). Chick-peas have a particularly satisfying flavor and are exceptional for their ability to retain their texture when canned, making them a highly rewarding convenience ingredient. You can add them to soups, salads, and vegetarian main dishes. They are rich in fiber, folate, protein, and complex carbohydrates.

chili powder Chili powder is a commercially prepared seasoning mixture made from ground dried chilies, oregano, cumin, coriander, salt, and dehydrated garlic, and sometimes cloves and allspice. Chili powders can range in strength from mild to very hot; if it's a chili

powder you've never tried before, give it a taste test first. Pure ground chili powder, without any added spices, is also available, though mostly in gourmet stores and from mail-order spice houses. The heat and flavor of a pure chili powder will depend on the type of chili used to make it. Some common powdered chilies include jalapeño, ancho, and pasilla.

chili sauce Chili sauce is a thick, ketchup-like condiment seasoned with chili peppers (or chili powder), garlic, and spices. Chili sauce is a convenient, flavorful option for "spiking" Mexican, Tex-Mex, Creole, and other spicy-hot dishes. Nutritionally, chili sauce is roughly equivalent to ketchup, and can be substituted for ketchup if you like the heat.

chutney Chutney is a fruit- or vegetable-based condiment typical of Indian cuisine. It can range from smooth to chunky, from sweet to sour, from spicy to mild. It can also be fresh or preserved. The most typical type of chutney sold in supermarkets is of the chunky, sweet-sour, preserved variety and is most commonly made with mangoes. Though chutney is thought of as an accompaniment to food, it also makes a good flavor addi-

tion to dishes such as burgers, meatloaf, salad dressings, sauces, soups, and stews.

cinnamon Cinnamon is the dried inner bark of a tropical evergreen tree, of which there are about 100 different species, all with similar aromatic properties. The two most commonly available varieties are Ceylonese cinnamon and Chinese cinnamon. Chinese cinnamon, which is actually from the bark of the cassia tree, is not considered a true cinnamon (species *Cinnamomum verum*). Grown in Southern China and other parts of Eastern Asia, cassia is a dark reddish color and stronger in flavor than its Ceylonese cousin (*Cinnamomum zeylancium*). Cassia is less expensive to process than true cinnamons and is the type of "cinnamon" most commonly sold in supermarkets—though it is sometimes blended with Ceylonese cinnamon.

coriander, ground The tiny, round, yellow-tan seeds of the coriander plant have no flavor resemblance to the plant's leaves (which are commonly called cilantro). Coriander comes both as whole seeds and ground. Pungently spicy, yet sweet and slightly citrusy, coriander is a key component in

THE SAVVY SHOPPER

curries and is often used in spice cakes and cookies.

cumin The seed of a plant in the parsley family, nutty-flavored whole or ground cumin seeds are often a component of chili powder; indeed, the spice is commonly used to flavor many Mexican and Tex-Mex dishes. Cumin is also a key ingredient in curry powder. To bring out its flavor, lightly toast cumin before adding it to a dish.

egg substitute There are two basic types of egg substitute commonly available in supermarkets. One is egg whites with some food coloring and flavors added so that the egg white mixture resembles beaten whole eggs. There is also an egg substitute that is merely egg whites. They are both refrigerated and can be found in the dairy department. Neither one has any cholesterol or fat. They are a convenient way to have just egg whites and no yolks (where all of the fat and cholesterol are) without having to separate real eggs. However, you do pay a price for this convenience. It costs about three times as much to use egg substitute as it would to buy real eggs and simply throw away the yolks.

ginger, ground Ground ginger is a "warm" spice made by drying and pulverizing gingerroot. A standard ingredient in spicy desserts, ginger is used in savory dishes as well as in baking. Ground ginger is not, however, a substitute for fresh ginger. Like all spices, ginger loses its flavor with time; buy a new jar if the ginger in your spice rack lacks a lively bite.

honey Honey is a convenient sweetener, especially in cold dishes, because you don't have to dissolve sugar over heat: The honeybee has already processed it for you. While insignificant in nutrients other than calories, honey can be found in assorted flavors (depending on where the bees gathered the nectar), styles, and colors. Honey should never be given to infants under 1 year as they lack certain stomach acids that would protect them against certain strains of botulin toxins, which may be present in honey. When measuring out honey, pour it into a measuring cup or spoon that has been sprayed with nonfat cooking spray as this prevents the honey from sticking to the utensil.

hot pepper sauce Once upon a time, if you told someone to buy hot pepper sauce, you could be confident that they

would come home with a red Louisiana-style hot sauce with the tang of vinegar. Now there is a world of hot sauces, with heat levels and blends of ingredients that vary considerably from one brand to another. There are, however, a couple of styles of hot sauce that are fairly consistent: For example, in addition to the red Louisiana-style sauces, there are green jalapeño-based sauces, Caribbean-style sauces (which are sweet-sour and often include fruit), and super-hot Jamaican hot sauces (which are yellow because they are made with yellow mustard and hot because they're made with Scotch Bonnet chili peppers). There are also garlicky Southeast Asian sauces.

ketchup Until recently, ketchup was a garden-variety American condiment. But with the publicity over the plant pigment called lycopene, which is believed to have healthful properties, ketchup—a good source of lycopene—has moved into the spotlight. This has resulted in a variety of flavored ketchups, but it has also meant the arrival of "no-salt-added" ketchup, which is a good compromise between the fairly high-sodium regular ketchup and the rather bland low-sodium ketchup.

mayonnaise Like many other high-fat foods, mayonnaise comes in several versions that have less fat than the standard product. For our recipes we have chosen to use the reduced-fat version (usually labeled "Light"), because although the fat-free and low-fat versions have less fat, they are oddly sweet.

milk, evaporated Evaporated milk is homogenized milk that has had much of its water removed, leaving behind a concentration of milk fat and solids. It has a slightly sweet taste because of the concentration of lactose (milk sugar), but it should not be confused with sweetened condensed milk, which has sugar added to it. Evaporated milk comes in a number of forms, depending on how much of the milk fat has been removed. There are regular (full-fat), low-fat (2%), and fat-free forms. Store at room temperature for up to 6 months until opened, then refrigerate for up to 1 week.

mushrooms, portobello Originally imported from Italy, but now widely grown in the United States, tan-skinned portobellos are actually fully mature cremini mushrooms. (Portobellos have gained such popularity that cremini are now often marketed as "baby bellas.") As large as 4 to 5 inches in diameter, portobellos are hearty, rather meaty-flavored mushrooms. They are sold with and without their fibrous stems, and unlike many other mushrooms, their black gills are completely exposed. Portobellos are now also sold presliced in shrink-wrapped packages in the produce department.

mustard, dijon Dijon mustard is a French-style prepared mustard made with dry white wine. Depending on the brand, the flavor of Dijon mustard can vary quite a bit, so try a few brands until you find a favorite.

oil, dark sesame The sesame oil most commonly found in supermarkets is a dark, polyunsaturated oil, pressed from toasted sesame seeds. Since it is often used in Asian cuisines, and because many brands of this oil have Asian-sounding names, cookbooks often refer to it as "Asian sesame oil," but in the store you will not find any labels that say this. The label is more likely to just say "sesame oil" or sometimes "roasted sesame oil." You will also find cold-pressed sesame oil in health-food stores; this type of oil is not from toasted sesame seeds, and is light in both flavor and color. The dark oil breaks down when heated, so it is not used for sautéing, but rather as a seasoning, added at the end of cooking.

orzo Orzo is a small pasta shape that resembles large grains of rice or unhulled barley (the Italian word *orzo* means barley). It's often used as a "soup pasta," which means tiny pasta shapes that cook up quickly in soups. Orzo can be served as a pasta dish, tossed with a sauce, or served as a simple side dish like rice.

paprika Paprika is a spice ground from a variety of red peppers and used in many traditional Hungarian and Spanish dishes. Paprika colors foods a characteristic brick-red and flavors dishes from sweet to spicy-hot, depending on the pepper potency. The most common type of supermarket paprika is sweet and mild, but you can also find Hungarian hot paprika. Since most recipes assume that you are using a sweet paprika, be careful not to use hot paprika in its place, since it can be as hot as chili powder or even cayenne.

peppers, jalapeño Jalapeño peppers are hot green chili peppers about two inches long and an inch in diameter, with rounded tips. Most of the heat resides in the membranes (ribs) of the pepper, so remove them for a milder effect—wear gloves to protect your hands from the volatile oils. Jalapeños are also sold pickled, whole or sliced. Although a really good fresh jalapeño has an incomparable flavor, there can be a wide range of heat; sometimes you'll get a fresh chili that has no more heat than a green bell pepper. Pickled jalapeños, on the other hand, are a reliable source of chili heat.

peppers, roasted Roasted peppers are a wonderful addition to soups, stews, and salads, and also make a good base for low-calorie salad dressings or pasta sauces. The peppers are first roasted to simplify peeling off their skins, and the roasting also cooks them so they are soft and flavorful. The peeled, roasted peppers are then packed in brine to preserve them. You can get both red and yellow peppers in this form. Rinsing them before adding them to dishes removes some of the brine.

pesto Pesto is a heady concoction of fresh basil, garlic, nuts (traditionally pine nuts), Parmesan, and olive oil. Though it can be exceptionally high in fat, you only need to use a little bit to infuse a dish with its pungent flavors. Look for pesto in refrigerated tubs where fresh pasta is sold.

pizza crust, prebaked Prebaked pizza crusts are certainly a boon to the busy cook. They come with a range of fat and sodium levels, depending on the brand. The best choice is to buy a brand with a thin crust so you can maximize the nutrition of the pizza you make by concentrating on healthful toppings and not worrying about the calories from a thick crust.

potatoes, instant Potato granules or potato flakes are merely dehydrated potatoes, and are a nutritious way to thicken such things as soups and sauces. (Of course, it is also a convenient way to make mashed potatoes.) When shopping for instant potatoes, read the ingredient list to be sure there is no added sodium or fat. Many instant potatoes, however, have various additives to preserve freshness and improve texture.

pumpkin, canned Canned pumpkin, often labeled "solid-pack pumpkin," is an unsweetened puree of cooked pumpkin (and not to be confused with canned pumpkin pie filling, which has added sugar and spices). It is a convenience for cooks who do not have hours to spend cooking fresh pumpkin down to a thick concentrate. Although most people have probably used pumpkin puree to make pies, this wonderfully nutritious ingredient (extremely high in beta carotene) can also be used in soups, quick breads, cakes, and sauces.

rosemary This herb comes from an evergreen shrub. Indeed, a branch of fresh rosemary looks like a small sprig of evergreen, and is just as fragrant. Unlike most herbs, the difference between the flavor of fresh and dried rosemary is slight. When using fresh rosemary, it's necessary to remove the needles from the stem, then chop and crush them thoroughly. Dried rosemary (which is just the needles) should be crushed or crumbled before being added to a dish.

sage This native Mediterranean herb is most familiar as a seasoning for poultry stuffing. Sold as whole leaves (fresh or dried), rubbed (crumbled), and ground, sage has a bold, rather musty flavor and aroma. Try it with any type of poultry, or with pork, veal, or ham. Or use it in cheese sauces; in bean or vegetable soups and seafood chowders; or with cooked mushrooms, lima beans, peas, tomatoes, or eggplant.

salsa Salsa, which just means "sauce" in Spanish, is most typically spicy. And far and away the commonest salsa available in supermarkets is a tomato-based sauce. Tomato salsas can be made with either uncooked or cooked tomatoes, and have varying degrees of chili-pepper heat, ranging from mild to medium to hot. There is no objective measurement for these heat levels, so you have to be familiar with the brand to know exactly how spicy they will be. The uncooked forms of salsa are ordinarily sold in plastic tubs and are refrigerated. They tend to be more watery than salsas made from cooked tomatoes, which are sold in jars and are not refrigerated.

sour cream Sour cream is a tart, thick dairy product made by treating cream with a lactic acid culture. Regular sour cream contains at least 18% milk fat by volume; reduced-fat sour cream contains about 4% fat; fat-free sour cream may have a little bit of fat (under 0.5 gram per serving is considered fat-free). In cooking, the reduced-fat version

can be substituted for regular sour cream. Use the fat-free with caution since it behaves differently, especially in baking. To avoid curdling, do not subject sour cream to high heat.

soy sauce Soy sauce is a condiment made from fermented soybeans, roasted grain (wheat, barley, or rice are common), and salt. Traditional soy sauce is quite high in sodium and should be used sparingly. Most supermarkets carry reduced-sodium (about one-third less sodium than the traditional) and "lite" (about 50% less sodium) versions. Just be careful if you shop for soy sauce in an Asian market, because there is a type of Chinese soy sauce called "Light," a designation that does not refer to sodium content but to a certain style of soy sauce. Chinese light soy sauce is actually higher in sodium than regular soy sauce.

tarragon Essential in French cooking, tarragon has a faint undertone of anise or licorice. Because it is so flavorful, the herb may overshadow other herbs, so use it with discretion. Tarragon is an excellent choice with shellfish, such as crab or shrimp, or with poached, baked, or broiled fish. It also complements poultry. Try it in a vinai-

grette or other salad dressing, and with potatoes, peas, asparagus, carrots, mushrooms, or tomatoes.

thyme This versatile herb, though quite strong in flavor, is compatible with many foods. Add a little to tomato sauces; vegetable soups and clam and other seafood chowders; beef stew or pot roast; lamb dishes; poultry stuffings; and cooked vegetables, such as summer squash or green beans.

tomatoes, canned diced Canned diced tomatoes are a wonderful compromise between canned whole tomatoes and tomato sauce. They are chopped fine enough to cook down to a sauce if need be, but they still retain some texture. There are also a number of seasoned diced tomatoes, with such added ingredients as basil, jalapeños, Italian herbs, Mexican spices, garlic, or onion.

tomatoes, grape These small tear-shaped tomatoes are very sweet and flavorful. They are especially useful when you want to add fresh tomato flavor to salads, soups, or stews. They are available year round and are a welcome ingredient in the winter when most other tomatoes have no flavor.

Leading Sources of

fiber

food	calories	fiber (g)
†Black beans, cooked, 1 cup	227	15.0
†Chick-peas, cooked, 1 cup	269	12.5
†Baby lima beans, cooked, 1 cup	189	10.8
†Green peas, cooked, 1 cup	134	8.8
Raspberries, 1 cup	60	8.4
Bulgur, cooked, 1 cup	151	8.2
Blackberries, 1 cup	75	7.6
†Baked sweet potato, with skin, 8 oz,	279	7.3
†Oat bran, ½ cup	116	7.2
†Dried figs, 3 medium	145	7.0
Dried pears, ½ cup	236	6.8
Artichoke, 1 medium	60	6.5
Whole-wheat pasta, cooked, 1 cup	174	6.3
Wheat bran, ¼ cup	31	6.2
†Dried plums (prunes), ½ cup	203	6.0
†Barley, cooked, 1 cup	193	6.0
†Dried apricots, ½ cup	155	5.9
Butternut squash, cooked, 1 cup	82	5.7
Baked potato, with skin, 8 oz	247	5.4
†Carrots, cooked, 1 cup	70	5.1
Buckwheat groats, cooked, 1 cup	155	4.5
†Hass avocado, ½ medium	153	4.2
Pear, 1 fresh	98	4.0
†Oatmeal, cooked, 1 cup	145	4.0
Blueberries, 1 cup	81	3.9
Almonds, roasted, 1 oz	166	3.9
Sunflower seeds, ¼ cup	205	3.8
†Apple, with skin, 1 medium	81	3.7
Wheat germ, toasted, ¼ cup	108	3.6
Brown rice, cooked, 1 cup	216	3.5
Strawberries, 1 cup	43	3.3
†Carrots, 1 cup grated raw	47	3.3
Mushrooms, cooked, 1 cup	48	2.4
Grapefruit, ½ medium	39	1.3

†Foods particularly high in soluble fiber.

calcium

food	calories	calcium (mg)
Tofu, firm (made with calcium sulfate), 3 oz	123	581
Yogurt, plain, fat-free, 1 cup	137	488
Yogurt, plain, low-fat, 1 cup	155	448
Milk, nonfat dry powder, ⅓ cup	109	411
Milk, fat-free, 1 cup	100	352
Parmesan cheese, 1 oz	111	335
Ricotta cheese, part-skim, ½ cup	170	335
Sardines, canned (with bones), 3 oz	177	325
Milk, low-fat (1%), 1 cup	102	300
Cheddar cheese, reduced-fat, 1 oz	81	253
Collard greens, cooked, 1 cup	49	226
Salmon, canned (with bones), 3 oz	130	203

folate

food	calories	folate (mcg)
Lentils, cooked, 1 cup	230	358
Black-eyed peas, cooked, 1 cup	200	358
Pinto beans, cooked, 1 cup	234	294
Chick-peas, cooked, 1 cup	269	282
Spinach, cooked, 1 cup	41	263
Asparagus, cooked, 1 cup	43	263
Black beans, cooked, 1 cup	227	256
Kidney beans, cooked, 1 cup	225	230
Green soybeans, cooked, 1 cup	254	200
Chicory, raw, chopped, 1 cup	41	198
Collard greens, cooked, 1 cup	49	177
Turnip greens, cooked, 1 cup	29	170
Romaine lettuce, chopped, 2 cups	16	152
Fortified oatmeal, cooked, 1 cup	105	151
Beets, diced, cooked, 1 cup	75	136
Split peas, cooked, 1 cup	231	127
Spinach, raw, chopped, 2 cups	13	116
Orange juice, 1 cup	112	109
Brussels sprouts, cooked, 1 cup	61	94
White rice, enriched, cooked, 1 cup	205	92

Recommended Intakes

The charts below provide the adult RDAs established by the National Academy of Sciences for vitamins and minerals. For some vitamins and minerals, not enough is known to recommend a specific amount; in these cases, the Academy has recommended a range called the Estimated Safe and Adequate Daily Dietary Intake. All values are for adults (over age 19).

vitamins

Vitamin A	
women	700 mcg
men	900 mcg
Vitamin C	
women	75 mg
men	90 mg
Vitamin D	
age 19-50	200 IU
age 51-70	400 IU
age 70+	600 IU
Vitamin E	15 mg
Vitamin K	
women	90 mcg
men	120 mcg
Thiamin	
women	1.1 mg
men	1.2 mg
Riboflavin	
women	1.1 mg
men	1.3 mg
Niacin	
women	14 mg
men	16 mg
Pantothenic acid	5 mg
Vitamin B_6	
women and men 19-50	1.3 mg
women 51+	1.5 mg
men 51+	1.7 mg
Vitamin B_{12}	2.4 mcg
Folate (folic acid)	400 mcg
Biotin	30 mcg

minerals

Calcium	
age 19-50	1,000 mg
age 51+	1,200 mg
Chloride	No RDA
Chromium	
women 19-50	25 mcg
women 51+	20 mcg
men 19-50	35 mcg
men 51+	30 mcg
Copper	900 mcg
Fluoride	
women	3 mg
men	4 mg
Iodine	150 mcg
Iron	
women 19-50	18 mg
women 51+	8 mg
men 19+	8 mg
Magnesium	
women 19-30	310 mg
women 31+	320 mg
men 19-30	400 mg
men 31+	420 mg
Manganese	
women	1.8 mg
men	2.3 mg
Molybdenum	45 mcg
Phosphorus	700 mg
Potassium	1,600 to 2,000 mg minimum
Selenium	55 mcg
Sodium	2,400 mg maximum
Zinc	
women	8 mg
men	11 mg

recipe index

recipe index

recipe index

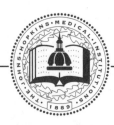

JOHN A. FLYNN, M.D., M.B.A., F.A.C.P, F.A.C.R., is a graduate of the University of Missouri-Columbia School of Medicine. He completed his medical residency and fellowship in rheumatology at Johns Hopkins Hospital, where he is now an associate professor in the Division of Molecular and Clinical Rheumatology and clinical director of the division of General Internal Medicine in the Department of Medicine.

His areas of research include investigating new ways to optimize therapy for spondylarthritis and looking into innovations for educating physicians-in-training in the outpatient setting. He was recently awarded the American College of Rheumatology's Clinician Scholar Education Award. He has published in journals such as *Arthritis & Rheumatism, Arthritis Care & Research*, and *The New England Journal of Medicine*, and is co-editor of the textbook, *Cutaneous Medicine*.

LORA BROWN WILDER, Sc.D., M.S., R.D., a registered dietitian, received her M.S. in nutrition from the University of Maryland and her Sc.D. in public health from Johns Hopkins University. She is currently an assistant professor at the Johns Hopkins School of Medicine, and is also affiliated with USDA and the University of Maryland's Department of Nutrition and Food Science. Dr. Wilder has served on various advisory committees related to nutrition, including the American Heart Association and the National Institutes of Health, and helped set up the first Johns Hopkins Preventive Cardiology Program.

In her research, Dr. Wilder has studied the effects of coffee on fatty acids and investigated behavioral strategies to reduce coronary risk factors. Her current research is in the area of dietary assessment methodology. She contributed to Nutritional Management: The Johns Hopkins Handbook and has been published in such journals as *Circulation, American Journal of Medicine*, and *Journal of the American Medical Association*.

SIMEON MARGOLIS, M.D., PH.D., a professor of medicine and biological chemistry at the Johns Hopkins University School of Medicine, is the medical editor for *The Johns Hopkins Medical Letter: Health After 50* and the consulting medical editor for *The Johns Hopkins Cookbook Library*.

The Johns Hopkins Cookbook Library is published by Medletter Associates, Inc.

Rodney Friedman Publisher

Kate Slate Executive Editor

Sandra Rose Gluck Test Kitchen Director, Food Editor

Timothy Jeffs Art Director

Maureen Mulhern-White Senior Writer

Patricia Kaupas Writer/Researcher

James W. Brown Associate Editor